AUTOIMMUNITY, RHEUMATOID ARTHRITIS AND CYCLOSPORIN A

(SANDIMMUN®)

AUTOIMMUNITY, RHEUMATOID ARTHRITIS AND CYCLOSPORIN A

(SANDIMMUN®)

Edited by

Y. Mizushima and B. Amor

The Proceedings of a Symposium held
at the XVIIth ILAR Congress of Rheumatology
Rio de Janeiro, September 1989

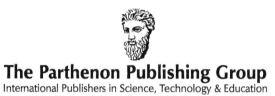

The Parthenon Publishing Group

International Publishers in Science, Technology & Education

Casterton Hall, Carnforth,
Lancs, LA6 2LA, UK

120 Mill Road, Park Ridge,
New Jersey, USA

Published in the UK and Europe by
The Parthenon Publishing Group Ltd.
Casterton Hall
Carnforth, Lancs. LA6 2LA

Published in North America by
The Parthenon Publishing Group Inc.
120 Mill Road
Park Ridge
New Jersey, NJ, USA

ISBN: 1-85070-305-1

Typeset by Lasertext Ltd., Stretford, Manchester
Printed and bound in Great Britain by
Butler & Tanner Ltd., Frome and London

Contents

List of principal contributors

B. Amor
Clinique de Rhumatologie
Hôpital Cochin
27, rue du Faubourg St. Jacques
F-75674 Paris Cedex 14
France

B.W. Kirkham
Rheumatology Unit
United Medical and Dental Schools
Guy's Hospital
London SE1 9RT
UK

Y. Mizushima
4-25-20, Daita
Setagaya-ku
Tokyo 155
Japan

M.-H. Pitty
Sandoz Pharma AG
Basle
Switzerland

E. del Pozo
Sandoz Research Institute
  Berne Ltd.
Monbijoustrasse 115
CH-3007 Berne
Switzerland

R.G.G. Russell
Department of Human Metabolism
  and Clinical Biochemistry
University of Sheffield Medical
  School
Sheffield S10 2RX
UK

W.E. Seaman
Veterans Administration Medical
  Center
Arthritis/Immunology Section
  (111R)
4150 Clement Street
San Francisco
CA 94121
USA

P. Tugwell
McMaster University
Department of Clinical
  Epidemiology and Biostatics
1200 Main Street West
Hamilton
Ontario L8N 3Z5
Canada

Introduction

Y. Mizushima

I have been asked by a Japanese pressman which are the five most important drugs developed recently? My answer was, 'They are H_2-blockers, prostaglandins, cyclosporin A, acyclovir and erythropoietin'. These drugs have new chemical structures and unique mechanisms in action. They stimulate the development of other drugs with similar modes of action. Most importantly, a great therapeutic jump has been achieved with these drugs.

Cyclosporin A (Sandimmun®) is a cyclic and lipophilic peptide. It selectively inhibits the production of interleukin 2 and other cytokines without interfering with normal cell proliferation, unlike other immunosuppressive drugs. It has led to marked progress in the field of solid organ transplantation.

Since interleukin 2 and other cytokines are required for the development of many autoimmune diseases in man, the application of cyclosporin A to these diseases and conditions has been tested. A double-blind trial conducted in Japan of cyclosporin A for the treatment of Behçet's disease clearly showed the effectiveness of the drug, and many studies on the application of cyclosporin A to immunological diseases have been published. As far as I know, however, the papers in this book are the first to overview the animal studies and the clinical efficacy and safety studies of cyclosporin A in rheumatoid arthritis.

Recent studies have shown that interleukin 2 and other cytokines modulate not only immune systems but also activities of the central nervous system and bone metabolites. The effects of cyclosporin A on bone metabolites are also described in this volume.

We hope that this volume on cyclosporin A stimulates further studies on immune systems, cyclosporin A and related compounds.

I

Autoimmunity: current concepts

W.E. Seaman

INTRODUCTION

The 1980s have brought substantial advancement in our knowledge of normal immune regulation. Progress in autoimmunity has been slower, in part because a central question in immune regulation has not yet been answered sufficiently well: how is immune tolerance to self-antigens established and sustained?

While we await the answer to this question, there are other questions that can be asked. This very brief introduction to the topic of autoimmunity will pose three of these questions:

(1) Is autoimmunity subject to normal mechanisms of immune regulation?

(2) Is the autoimmune response mediated by distinct subsets of T cells or B cells?

(3) Is autoimmunity antigen-driven?

IS AUTOIMMUNITY SUBJECT TO NORMAL MECHANISMS OF IMMUNE REGULATION?

The generation of a normal antibody response to most protein antigens requires three cells: B cells, T cells, and specialized antigen-presenting cells (usually macrophages) (Figure 1). The production of most autoantibodies appears to require not only B cells but also T cells. The evidence for

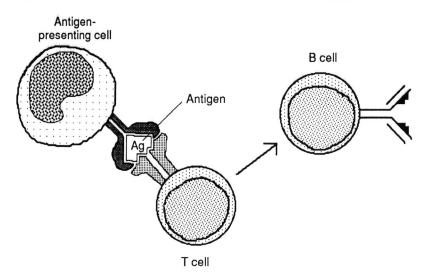

Figure 1 The three cells required for a normal antibody response to most protein antigens. In this simplified diagram, a T cell recognizes antigen on specialized antigen-presenting cells and then provides help to B cells, which produce antibody

this comes primarily from studies in mice. For example, David Wofsy and I have studied NZB/NZW mice, a model for human lupus erythematosus. By treatment with monoclonal antibodies against murine CD4 (mCD4), these mice could be depleted of T 'helper' cells. Treatment of NZB/NZW mice early in life prevented autoimmunity[1]. Treatment of mice after the onset of autoimmunity reversed it. Carteron and colleagues demonstrated that treatment of NZB/NZW mice with F(ab′)$_2$ anti-mCD4 also blocked autoimmunity[2]. In the treated mice, circulating T cells were coated with F(ab′)$_2$ anti-mCD4, but the T cells were not depleted. Thus the effects of anti-mCD4 on immunity were not dependent on depletion of CD4+ target cells. Similar treatment has produced beneficial results in a variety of autoimmune diseases in mice, including non-obese diabetic mice[3], collagen-induced arthritis[4], experimental autoimmune encephalomyelitis[5] and experimental myasthenia gravis[6]. Thus, T cells may be required for a variety of autoimmune diseases.

Does the activation of T cells have the same requirements for autoimmune responses as for normal immune responses? Figure 2 provides a schematic illustration of the molecular interactions that permit the activation of CD4+ T cells in response to foreign antigen on

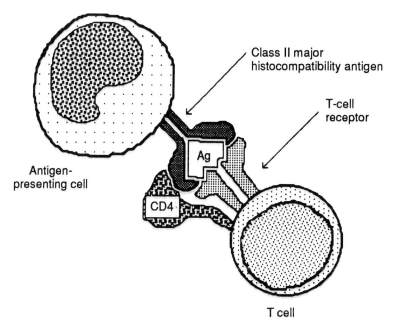

Figure 2 A closer look at the interaction between antigen-presenting cells and T 'helper cells'. Foreign antigen is bound to a class II major histocompatibility antigen. This complex is recognized by the T-cell receptor. The interaction is strengthened by the non-specific binding of CD4 to the class II major histocompatibility antigen

antigen-presenting cells. On the surface of antigen-presenting cells, the foreign antigen is bound to major histocompatibility antigens[7]. For the response by CD4 + T cells this must be a class II major histocompatibility antigen, i.e. HLA-DP, HLA-DQ, or HLA-DR[8]. The complex of antigen plus major histocompatibility antigen is recognized by the T-cell antigen receptor, and this interaction provides signals for the initiation of T-cell activation. The activation of T cells is greatly enhanced by an additional interaction, the binding of CD4 to the class II major histocompatibility antigen[8].

The inhibition of autoimmunity by F(ab')$_2$ antibodies to CD4 suggests (but does not prove) that CD4 may participate in the response of autoimmune T cells as well as normal cells. Similarly, the association of autoimmune diseases with specific alleles of the class II major histocompatibility antigens (e.g. the association of rheumatoid arthritis with HLA-DR4) suggests that the activation of autoimmune T cells may utilize subsets of class II major histocompatibility antigen. Whether this role for the class II major histocompatibility antigen is the same as its role in the presentation of foreign antigens is unknown.

IS THE AUTOIMMUNE RESPONSE MEDIATED BY SUBSETS OF T CELLS OR B CELLS?

If the autoimmune response were mediated by subsets of T or B cells, and if these could be distinguished from the cells that are required for an immune response to foreign antigens, it might be possible to selectively inhibit autoimmunity without reducing normal immunity. From the studies cited above, it appears that most autoimmune responses may be dependent on CD4+ cells. CD4+ cells are also required for most antibody responses to foreign protein antigens. Normal cellular immunity, however, can persist in the absence of functional CD4+ cells, albeit with reduced strength.

Is autoimmunity mediated by subsets of CD4+ T cells? Subsets of CD4+ T cells have been defined on the basis of function, surface phenotype, and by selective utilization of genes that encode the T-cell antigen receptor.

At the functional level, Mossman and colleagues demonstrated that cloned CD4+ T cell lines could usually be divided into one of two types: one type produced relatively large amounts of interferon-γ (IFN-γ) and interleukin-2 (IL-2), while the other produced relatively large amounts of IL-4, IL-5 and IL-6[9]. It is not yet established that these functional distinctions are characteristic of T cells *in vivo*. These *in vitro* findings, nonetheless, underscore the point that inhibition of one T-cell function may not inactivate another. This is especially relevant to the treatment of autoimmunity. It would be advantageous if some T-cell functions could be preserved while others are expressed. It is also possible, however, that attempts to suppress autoimmunity through one functional T-cell pathway may be inadequate or misdirected.

Several surface markers can distinguish subsets of T cells that appear to correlate with the state of T-cell activation. For example, subsets of T cells express different isoforms of the CD45 (T200) antigen. Un-primed T cells express isoforms of 205–220 kDa, called CD45R. Among CD4+ T cells, exposure to antigen and the development of help for B cells is associated with a switch to an isoform of 180 kDa, called

CD45RO, identified by the monoclonal antibody UCHL1[10,11]. The T cells that accumulate in rheumatoid synovium express predominantly CD45RO, providing a possible target for immunotherapy[12]. Such therapy, however, would presumably impair normal immunity as well as autoimmunity, and it would not be restricted to effects on CD4+ cells; CD8+ cells also express the various isoforms of CD45.

T-cell activation leads to expression of the p55 component of the IL-2 receptor (IL-2R, TAC antigen)[13]. This provides another potential target for immune suppression[14]. Interestingly, however, T cells in the rheumatoid synovium express only low levels of this activation antigen[15].

T cells might also be subdivided by the restricted use of variable region genes to form the T-cell antigen receptor, analogous to restricted idiotypes on immunoglobulins. With regard to restricted use of T-cell antigen receptors by autoimmune T cells, only limited information is yet available. In experimental autoimmune encephalomyelitis, where the autoimmune T-cell response to myelin basic protein is highly limited in specificity, some (but not all) mouse strains rely entirely on the use of Vβ8 to produce the T-cell antigen receptor that recognizes the antigen[16]. For these mice, treatment with a monoclonal antibody directed against receptors encoded by Vβ8 protects against disease[16]. In rats, experimental autoimmune encephalomyelitis can be prevented by immunizing animals against clones of T cells that respond specifically to myelin basic protein[17]. In collagen-induced arthritis, such restricted use of T-cell receptor genes has not been identified, but immunization against T-cell lines that recognize type II collagen can similarly protect against disease[18].

Turning from T cells to B cells, the latter clearly make restricted use of variable region genes for generating antibodies against a variety of autoantigens, even when the antigens are relatively complex. For example, both in humans with systemic lupus erythematosus and in NZB/NZW mice, the bulk of anti-DNA antibodies may be accounted for by a few immunoglobulin idiotypes[19,20].

In NZB mice, a parent of NZB/NZW mice, it has been proposed that production of autoantibodies is initiated primarily within the minority of B cells that express CD5, an antigen normally found on T cells[21,22]. This is a controversial area. IgG autoantibodies, which predominate in most severe autoimmune diseases, cannot come from

CD5+ B cells which produce only IgM antibodies. It is possible that CD5+ B cells serve as precursors for such cells, but this has not been directly demonstrated.

A substantial portion of CD5+ B cells appear committed to the production of IgM rheumatoid factors[23]. Likewise, among chronic B-cell lymphocytic leukemias, virtually all of which express CD5, a high proportion make rheumatoid factors. Of considerable interest is the demonstration that IgM rheumatoid factors, produced either by normal cells or by malignant cells, are encoded by germ-line immunoglobulin genes, i.e. they have not undergone somatic mutation. This is not due to lack of stimulation; the production of IgM rheumatoid factors is detectable in normal B cells and is increased during infection. These observations demonstrate the normal regulation (as opposed to mere suppression) of an autoimmune response, and they indicate that such regulation includes the prevention of somatic mutations in rheumatoid factors, or their selective removal. In rheumatoid arthritis, however, this response expands, rheumatoid factors become increasingly poly-clonal, and IgG rheumatoid factors appear.

IS THE AUTOIMMUNE RESPONSE ANTIGEN-DRIVEN?

The evidence that autoimmunity has many of the same requirements as a normal immune response – and that autoimmunity may be governed by many of the same rules – supports the contention that autoimmunity may be generated in response to a specific antigen. Moreover, auto-immune diseases can be stimulated by specific infections, such as streptococcal pharyngitis or enteric infection with certain strains of *Shigella, Salmonella, Yersinia* or *Campylobacter.*

On the other hand, non-specific stimuli can lead to autoimmunity, as in the activation of B cells by allogeneic T cells during a graft-versus-host reaction. In NZB/NZW mice, Steinberg and his colleagues have argued that the initial autoimmune T-cell response is similarly non-specific[24]. In both the graft-versus-host reaction and in NZB/NZW mice, however, the autoimmune response eventually becomes highly restricted. In NZB/NZW mice, with advanced disease, Steinberg and colleagues provide evidence that the disease may become antigen-driven, because the autoimmune response, but not the response to a foreign antigen, is sustained following the transfer of lymphocytes to a syngeneic host.

In reactive arthritis following enteric infections, Granfors and colleagues have demonstrated the reaction of anti-*Yersinia* antibodies with synovial fluid inflammatory cells, indicating the presence of bacterial antigens within the joint[25]. With chronic disease, however, these can no longer be detected. Thus, even if autoimmunity is antigen-driven, the initial reponse to a foreign antigen may be sustained despite the loss of the original antigenic stimulus – perhaps by the initiation of a response to a self-antigen.

CONCLUSION

This brings us back to the central question in immunology. How is immune tolerance to self established and maintained? Turning to the model provided in Figure 1, immune tolerance could be regulated at the level of B cells, T cells or antigen-presenting cells. There is evidence in favor of all these possibilities, but it is clear that the primary focus for immune regulation is through T cells. This regulation includes both negative selection of self-reactive T cells during development and the further restriction of autoimmune responses in the mature host. We are in the midst of rapid growth in our understanding of T-cell development in the thymus. Less is known about the regulation of mature T cells. Each new understanding, however, offers the opportunity for the development of new methods for immune regulation and, perhaps, for the prevention of autoimmunity.

The participation of the author was sponsored by the Scientific Committee of the ILAR Congress.

REFERENCES

1. Wofsy, D. and Seaman, W.E. (1985). Successful treatment of autoimmunity in NZB/NZW F$_1$ mice with monoclonal antibody to L3T4. *J. Exp. Med.,* **161**, 378–91
2. Carteron, N.L., Schimenti, C.L. and Wofsy, D. (1989). Treatment of

murine lupus with F(ab')$_2$ fragments of monoclonal antibody to L3T4: suppression of autoimmunity does not depend on T helper cell depletion. *J. Immunol.*, **142**, 1470–5

3. Koike, T., Itoh, Y., Ishi, T., Ito, I., Takabayashi, K., Maruyama, N., Tomioka, H. and Yoshido, S. (1987). Preventive effect of monoclonal anti-L3T4 antibody on development of diabetes in NOD mice. *Diabetes*, **36**, 539–41

4. Ranges, G.E., Sriram, S. and Cooper, S.M. (1985). Prevention of type II collagen-induced arthritis by *in vivo* treatment with anti-L3T4. *J. Exp. Med.*, **162**, 1105–10

5. Waldor, M.K., Sriram, S., Hardy, R., Herzenberg, L.A., Lanier, L., Lim, M. and Steinman, L. (1985). Reversal of experimental allergic encephalomyelitis with monoclonal antibody to a T-cell subset marker. *Science*, **227**, 415–17

6. Christados, P. and Dauphinée, M.J. (1986). Immunotherapy for myasthenia gravis: a murine model. *J. Immunol.*, **136**, 2437–40

7. Pernis, B., Silverstein, S.C. and Vogel, H. (eds.) (1988). *Processing and Presentation of Antigens.* (New York: Academic Press)

8. Bierer, B.E., Sleckman, B.P., Ratnofsky, S.E. and Burakoff, S.J. (1989). The biological roles of CD2, CD4 and CD8 in T-cell activation. In Paul, W., Fathman, C.G. and Metzger, H. (eds.) *Ann. Rev. Immunol.*, **7**, 579–99

9. Mossman, T.R. and Coffman, R.L. (1989). TH1 and TH2 cells: different patterns of lymphokine secretion lead to different functional properties. In Paul, W., Fathman, C.G. and Metzger, H. (eds.) *Ann. Rev. Immunol.*, **7**, 145–73

10. Clement, L.T., Yamashita, N. and Martin, A.M. (1988). The functionally distinct subpopulations of human CD4+ helper/inducer T lymphocytes defined by anti-CD45R antibodies derive sequentially from a differentiation pathway that is regulated by activation-dependent post-thymic differentiation. *J. Immunol.*, **141**, 1463–70

11. Terry, L.A., Brown, M.H. and Beverly, P.C. (1988). The monoclonal antibody, UCHL1, recognizes a 180 000 MW component of the human leukocyte-common antigen, CD45. *Immunology*, **64**, 331–6

12. Moore, K., Walters, M.T., Jones, D.B., Garvey, E., Harvey, J., Cawley, M.I. and Smith, J.L. (1988). An immunohistochemical study of CD45+ lymphocyte subsets within inflammatory lesions with special reference to rheumatoid arthritis and inflammatory bowel disease. *Immunology*, **65**, 457–63

13. Waldmann, T.A. (1989). The multi-subunit interleukin-2 receptor. *Ann. Rev. Biochem.*, **58**, 875–911

14. Strom, T.B. and Kelley, V.E. (1989). Toward more selective therapies to block undesired immune responses. *Kidney Int.*, **35**, 1026–33

15. Pitzalis, C., Kingsley, G., Lanchbury, J.S., Murphy, J. and Panayi, G.S. (1987). Expression of HLA-DR, DQ and DP antigens and interleukin-2 receptor on synovial fluid T lymphocyte subsets in rheumatoid arthritis: evidence for 'frustrated' activation. *J. Rheumatol.*, **14**, 662–6

16. Acha-Orbea, H., Mitchell, D.J., Timmermann, L., Wraith, D.C., Tausch, G.S., Waldor, M.K., Zamvil, S.S., McDevitt, H.O. and Steinman, L. (1988). Limited heterogeneity of T cell receptors from lymphocytes mediating autoimmune encephalomyelitis allows specific immune intervention. *Cell,* **54**, 263–73

17. Cohen, I.R. (1986). Regulation of autoimmune disease: physiological and therapeutic. *Immunol. Rev.*, **943**, 5–21

18. Brahn, E. and Trentham, D.E. (1987). Attenuation of collagen arthritis and modulation of delayed-type hypersensitivity by type II collagen reactive T-cell lines. *Cell. Immunol.*, **109**, 139–47

19. Macworth, Y.C. and Schwartz, R.S. (1988). Autoantibodies to DNA. *C.R.C. Crit. Rev. Immunol.*, **8**, 147–73

20. Hahn, B.H. and Ebling, F.M. (1987). Idiotype restriction in murine lupus; high frequency of three public idiotypes on serum IgG in nephritic NZB/NZW F$_1$ mice. *J. Immunol.*, **138**, 2110–18

21. Hayakawa, K., Hardy, R.R., Honda, M., Herzenberg, L.A., Steinberg, A.D. and Herzenberg, L.A. (1984). Ly-1 B cells: functionally distinct lymphocytes that secrete IgM autoantibodies. *Proc. Natl. Acad. Sci. USA,* **81**, 2494–8

22. Hayakawa, K. and Hardy, R.R. (1988). Normal, autoimmune, and malignant CD5 + B cells: the Ly-1 B lineage? *Ann. Rev. Immunol.*, **6**, 197–218

23. Carson, D.A., Chen, P.P., Fox, R.I., Kipps, T.J., Jirik, F., Goldfien, R.D., Silverman, G., Radoux, V. and Fong, S. (1987). Rheumatoid factors and immune networks. *Ann. Rev. Immunol.*, **5**, 109–26

24. Klinman, D.M. and Steinberg, A.D. (1987). Systemic autoimmune disease arises from polyclonal B cell activation. *J. Exp. Med.*, **165**, 1755–60

25. Granfors, K., Jalkanen, S., von-Essen, R., Lahesmaa-Rantala, R., Isomaki, O., Pekkola-Heina, K., Merilahti-Palo, R., Saario, R., Isomaki, H. and Toivanen, A. (1989). Yersinia antigens in synovial-fluid cells from patients with reactive arthritis. *N. Engl. J. Med.*, **320**, 216–21

2

Laboratory measures of disease activity in rheumatoid arthritis

B.W. Kirkham and G.S. Panayi

INTRODUCTION

A considerable amount of effort has been and is being devoted to the development of laboratory measures of rheumatoid disease activity. There are two principal aims behind this effort: first, to predict outcome of disease in individual patients and, second, to screen drugs of potential disease remitting power. This brief review outlines and discusses work to date in this important and rapidly developing area of rheumatological research.

ACUTE PHASE RESPONSE

Major increases in the plasma concentrations of a group of proteins, called the acute phase proteins, occur within 24–72 hours of an inflammatory stimulus, as part of the body's response to tissue injury or infection. This response also leads to changes in other serum constituents such as a rise in very low density lipoprotein and triglyceride, a fall in high density lipoproteins, and a fall in the concentration of zinc and iron[1]. In humans, the major acute phase proteins are C-reactive protein and serum amyloid A protein. The most widely used laboratory measures of the acute phase response in clinical medicine are measurements of the erythrocyte sedimentation rate and C-reactive protein concentration[2].

Erythrocyte sedimentation rate

It was known by the early Greeks that the sedimentation rate was elevated in disease states and the erythrocyte sedimentation rate has been in use for about 60 years[2]. The erythrocyte sedimentation rate is an indirect measure of increased concentrations of serum proteins, particularly asymmetrical molecules such as fibrinogen, which increase the charge dissipation characteristics of serum (the dielectric constant). This dissipation of electrical charge reduces the repulsive effects of the surface electrical field on red blood cells (the zeta potential) and allows the cohesive effects of the surface free energy (van der Waals forces) to predominate and aggregation results[3]. This aggregation can be visualized as rouleaux formation. Although fibrinogen is the most potent promoter of aggregation, elevations of other acute phase proteins and immuno-globulins also promote an elevation in the erythrocyte sedimentation rate[4].

Other factors that affect the erythrocyte sedimentation rate are anemia which gives a spurious increase in the erythrocyte sedimentation rate and changes in the shape and size of red blood cells (e.g. anisocytosis, microcytosis, spherocytosis) which reduce the erythrocyte sedimentation rate[5]. However, corrections for anemia are not now generally made. Changes in the normal levels of erythrocyte sedimentation rate in relation to age were thought to occur. Plasma viscosity provides a measure of similar serum changes as the erythrocyte sedimentation rate without red blood cell corrections[6]. However, the ease of erythrocyte sedimentation rate estimation has outweighed this theoretical advantage.

C-reactive protein

Unlike the erythrocyte sedimentation rate, C-reactive protein is a single acute phase protein. C-reactive protein was originally detected in human serum because of its ability to precipitate with the somatic C-polysaccharide of the pneumococcus in the presence of ionic calcium[7]. C-reactive protein is an aggregate of five identical non-covalently linked subunits arranged in cyclic symmetry[8]. The biological activity of C-reactive protein is unclear although it is thought to have an important biological role as C-reactive protein structure is highly conserved in many species from man to crab[2]. Levels of C-reactive protein rise rapidly within hours of an acute inflammatory stimulus as a result of increased hepatocyte synthesis[9]. The magnitude of the rise, which may reach 1000 times normal, is thought to be proportional to the extent of the inflammatory stimulus and persists in chronic inflammatory states. If the inflammatory stimulus remits, C-reactive protein levels begin to fall within hours[10]. Although initial assessment of C-reactive protein was only semiquantitative, the development of radial and electroimmuno-diffusion techniques provided quantitative results, and now immuno-assays are being used which give quantitative results and are simple and rapid to perform[11].

Control of acute phase protein synthesis

Hepatocyte synthesis of acute phase proteins has been investigated *in vitro* using murine or human liver cell lines. The most potent stimuli for those proteins are the cytokines interleukin 1, interleukin 6 and tumor necrosis factor α[12]. One of the early biological activities found to be interleukin 6 was called hepatocyte stimulating factor. In mouse and human cell lines, different cytokines preferentially stimulate some acute phase proteins and act additively or synergistically on others[13,14]. Baumann and colleagues[15], using human hepatoma cells, showed that interleukin 6 stimulated fibrinogen, haptoglobin and α_1-antitrypsin synthesis. Interleukin 1 induced a smaller increase in α_1-acid glycoprotein, haptoglobin and α_1-antichymotrypsin. They also found that dexamethasone enhanced the response to these cytokines without causing a direct effect alone. This effect of glucocorticoids has also been noted in murine models[13].

Acute phase proteins and rheumatoid arthritis

The erythrocyte sedimentation rate is the most widely used laboratory index of disease activity in rheumatoid arthritis. Although it has been suggested that plasma viscosity or C-reactive protein may be better[16,17], this is controversial[18]. The erythrocyte sedimentation rate and C-reactive protein have been found to decrease after treatment with disease modifying antirheumatic drugs[16]. This ability of disease modifying antirheumatic drugs to lower the erythrocyte sedimentation rate and/or

C-reactive protein levels as well as improving clinical indices is an important part of the definition of such a group of drugs[19]. Duthie and colleagues found that consecutive erythrocyte sedimentation rate values gave an indication of eventual functional capacity[20]. This result has been supported by Sherrer and colleagues[21]. However, other studies have found differing results[22,23]. Several authors have investigated the relationship between changes in erythrocyte sedimentation rate and C-reactive protein in response to treatment and changes in radiological disease progress. Scott and colleagues found the erythrocyte sedimentation rate to be related to radiological progression[24] and this result was supported by Sjoblom and colleagues[25].

Two studies have now shown that acute phase response levels are related to prognosis. Amos and colleagues studied 56 patients with stable erythrocyte sedimentation rate and C-reactive protein values despite treatment[26]. Over a period of 12 months they found that the development of erosions was lowest in the patients with a low erythrocyte sedimentation rate and C-reactive protein. They found little difference between erythrocyte sedimentation rate and C-reactive protein in predicting radiological outcome. Dawes and colleagues showed that if disease modifying antirheumatic drugs can suppress erythrocyte sedimentation rate and C-reactive protein, progressive radiological damage is prevented[27]. The question whether disease modifying antirheumatic drugs can significantly improve long-term outcome in terms of radiographic progression is still hotly debated.

Other acute phase reactants

Serum amyloid A protein levels are known to be elevated in patients with rheumatoid arthritis. Serum amyloid A protein is an apolipoprotein which can increase by a factor of 100–1000 in response to inflammatory stimuli[28]. It has been suggested by two groups that serum amyloid A protein may provide a more sensitive indicator of disease activity than the erythrocyte sedimentation rate or C-reactive protein[29,30]. However, the changes of serum amyloid A protein correlated closely with C-reactive protein and erythrocyte sedimentation rate in most patients and so any advantages are small. The disadvantages of serum amyloid A protein are the limited availability of a widely used serum amyloid A protein standard and a poorly defined normal range[30].

Ceruloplasmin levels are elevated in rheumatoid arthritis but the increase is only 2-fold. It is also elevated in women taking the oral contraceptive[31]. Haptoglobin levels are elevated in rheumatoid arthritis but less reliably than C-reactive protein. Haptoglobin is also complicated by having three common phenotypes and although rheumatoid arthritis patients have the same frequency of these phenotypes as controls, this measure is seldom used[19]. Dawes and colleagues found that changes in α_1-antitrypsin levels correlated with C-reactive protein levels in rheumatoid arthritis patients treated with disease modifying anti-rheumatic drugs[32].

Non-acute phase protein disease indicators

Histidine

Patients with active rheumatoid arthritis have been found to have low serum histidine levels which correlate well with acute phase protein levels. Gerber found that these levels were proportional to disease activity measured by a combination of clinical (grip strength, walking time, duration of stiffness) and laboratory (erythrocyte sedimentation rate, hematocrit, Latex rheumatoid factor) measurements, despite disease modifying antirheumatic drug treatment[33]. Pickup and colleagues measured serum histidine levels longitudinally after disease modifying antirheumatic drug treatment (gold, D-penicillamine, hydroxychloro-quine and prednisolone) and found that, despite clinical improvement, histidine levels changed only with D-penicillamine therapy[34]. Dixon showed that serum histidine levels increased significantly and in parallel to improvements in the articular index in patients treated with D-penicillamine and sulphasalazine, and increased, but not significantly, in patients treated with gold and hydroxychloroquine[19]. Gerber and Gerber reported that this isolated amino acid abnormality has a high degree of specificity for rheumatoid arthritis[35]. However, other groups have found conflicting results, with low serum histidine levels occurring in many arthropathies including osteoarthritis[36].

Sulphydryl

Total serum sulphydryl levels are low in rheumatoid arthritis, and have been shown to increase towards normal with clinical improvement[37] and after treatment with certain drugs[38]. Dixon showed that serum sulphydryl levels increased significantly in rheumatoid arthritis patients treated with D-penicillamine and azathioprine over a 6-month period[19]. The rise with D-penicillamine was in parallel with an improvement in the articular index which did not improve significantly with azathioprine. In patients with recent onset polyarthritis, low sulphydryl levels were found to be a good predictor of persisting rheumatoid arthritis[39].

Neutrophil activation markers

Cytidine deaminase is released from cytoplasmic granules of neutrophils and serum levels have been shown to correlate with clinical and conventional laboratory measures in rheumatoid arthritis[40]. When serial measurements of cytidine deaminase were made in a group of rheumatoid arthritis patients who had a flare of disease induced by stopping non-steroidal anti-inflammatory drug medication, serum levels rose within 2 days, before the clinical disease became worse. However, these increased levels were only transient and fell back to baseline levels within 2 days, despite continued clinical disease activity[41].

Leukocyte elastase is released from neutrophil azurophilic granules and in rheumatoid arthritis serum levels have been shown to correlate with clinical and laboratory indicators of disease activity[42].

Cartilage metabolism

Hyaline cartilage is mainly composed of proteoglycan and collagen. Type II collagen is found only in hyaline cartilage. Several groups have investigated the measurement of cartilage constituents as a way of assessing cartilage breakdown and disease activity. Saxne and colleagues measured synovial fluid proteoglycan fragments by an ELISA technique[43], in rheumatoid arthritis patients before and after intra-articular triamcinolone injections. They found stable levels over a 5-day period which then fell dramatically after triamcinolone treatment and, in one case, after spontaneous disease remission. This group also measured synovial fluid proteoglycan fragments taken from the knee of patients with rheumatoid arthritis and compared the levels with radiological changes 9–10 years later. They found a strong correlation between elevated levels and destructive radiological changes[44]. The source of these proteoglycan fragments is, however, not clear as fragments could be released from degraded cartilage or newly synthesized by synovial cells.

Urinary glycosaminoglycan and hydroxyproline excretion have been investigated as markers of cartilage degradation. Urinary levels of low molecular weight glycosaminoglycan are elevated in active rheumatoid arthritis[45]. However, the problem of whether the source of glycosamino-glycan is from cartilage breakdown or new synthesis has not been resolved.

Complement component C1q

Ochi and colleagues measured serum C1q levels by single radial immunodiffusion in 54 rheumatoid arthritis patients over a 5-year period[46]. They found three groups of patients. Some patients, who had all suffered rheumatoid arthritis for more than 7 years and who were clinically termed 'burned out' because of the absence of synovitis, had levels of C1q similar to healthy controls. Patients with 'active' disease had elevated C1q levels irrespective of erythrocyte sedimentation rates or C-reactive protein levels, in some cases without clinical synovitis. Patients with serum C1q levels greater than 250 µg/ml had sustained elevations of C-reactive proteins and had more new erosions on serial radiographs than patients with 'active disease' with C1q levels less than 250 µg/ml. In a subsequent report, Ochi and colleagues found similar results in a group of 240 patients followed for 10–15 years[47]. The C1q level in patients with a high number of eroded joints remained consistently above 250 µg/ml during the first 5 years of disease and declined gradually thereafter.

The prognostic significance of C1q has been questioned by Mottonen and colleagues who studied 60 rheumatoid arthritis patients with early disease[48]. They measured C1q levels at the beginning of the study and followed patients for 2 years. They found a difference between rheumatoid arthritis patients and healthy controls. However, only a small difference between patients who did not develop any erosions and those who developed 1–6 eroded joints was found ($p = 0.046$), and there was no difference between patients without erosions and those with six or more joints with erosions.

There were two main differences between these studies. Of the patients studied by Mottonen and colleagues, 59/60 received disease modifying antirheumatic drug therapy whereas Ochi and colleagues excluded these patients. Mottonen's group also found much lower C1q levels in the rheumatoid arthritis group compared to Ochi's group, although values for healthy control subjects were similar. Thus, the prognostic relevance of C1q in rheumatoid arthritis is unclear at present.

Comparative studies

Two studies have compared the use of many of the above laboratory measures in rheumatic disease. Bull and his group used a new analytical technique of consensus analysis to assess 31 laboratory measurements made monthly in 17 patients with rheumatoid arthritis treated with sulphasalazine for 7 months[49]. The results of 16 of these tests, which were found to be abnormal, i.e. they may be potential disease activity markers, were then rank ordered and the correlation between each test value and the consensus of all other test values for each patient on each visit was evaluated. The test with the poorest correlation was identified and those data eliminated and the procedure was repeated. This process allowed the identification of groups of tests with very close correlation (test families), which would appear to be measuring the same or very similar changes. The test families identified were C-reactive protein and orosomucoid; serum viscosity, plasma viscosity and globulin; and erythrocyte sedimentation rate, fibrinogen and zeta sedimentation ratio. One of these families was then compared to a consensus of the members of the other two families, to estimate the ability of that test to respond to aspects of rheumatoid arthritis that are measured by test families other than the one to which the test being evaluated belongs. In this estimation the erythrocyte sedimentation rate was consistently highest, followed by plasma viscosity, orosomucoid, zeta sedimentation rate, C-reactive protein, fibrinogen, globulin and, lastly, serum viscosity. This analysis has not correlated laboratory tests to clinical indices but has potential in identifying tests that either measure different aspects of the disease process, i.e. the test families, or in identifying the best screening tests, in this case the erythrocyte sedimentation rate.

The other comparative study, by Sitton and colleagues, compared levels of different laboratory disease indicators in different arthropathies[36]. They estimated C-reactive protein, plasma viscosity, serum histidine and total serum sulphydryl in 259 patients with rheumatoid arthritis, 84 patients with ankylosing spondylitis, 76 with osteoarthritis, 69 with psoriatic arthritis, 34 with systemic lupus erythematosus, 36 with Reiters syndrome and 121 normal controls. The rheumatoid arthritis group had the highest percentage of abnormal results for plasma viscosity, serum histidine, C-reactive protein and serum sulphydryl concentrations. The other arthropathies were all characterized by a lower incidence of abnormal results. Histidine levels were lowest in systemic lupus erythematosus, but were also low in rheumatoid arthritis and other arthropathies, negating the claims of Gerber and Gerber that this abnormality may be specific for rheumatoid arthritis[35]. Sulphydryl levels were lowest in the rheumatoid arthritis group but were lower than normal in osteoarthritis, ankylosing spondylitis, systemic lupus erythematosus and psoriatic arthritis. Levels of C-reactive protein were low in patients with systemic lupus erythematosus, confirming previous reports. C-reactive protein levels were elevated in 88% of ankylosing spondylitis patients.

Conclusion

The laboratory measures of disease activity discussed above can be broadly divided into two groups. The first group of acute phase proteins and other biochemical indicators of inflammation is the result of processes such as interleukin 1, tumor necrosis factor α and interleukin 6 induction of hepatic acute phase protein synthesis, while the mechanisms controlling other factors, such as reduced histidine levels, are unknown. Despite the existence of many options in this group, the erythrocyte sedimentation rate and C-reactive protein remain the most widely used measures of inflammation. The other options have not become clinically useful, as many measure very similar biological activities[49], and their proposed advantages are not great enough to displace the existing well-established and investigated measures. One exception to this may be sulphydryl determinations which may have prognostic value in early inflammatory arthritis[39]. The other main group attempts to monitor the consequences of the disease process by measuring degradation products of synovial compartment constituents, such as proteoglycan fragments.

CELL-MEDIATED IMMUNE MEASURES

Cell-mediated immune events are thought to play an important part in the continuing synovial inflammation of rheumatoid arthritis[50,51]. However, there have been few methods available to assess activity of this arm of the immune system. Emery and colleagues reported that 30–50% of patients with rheumatoid arthritis had a depressed response to recall antigens, demonstrated by skin testing and *in vitro* lymphocyte proliferation to tuberculin purified protein derivative[52]. This 'anergic' state did not correlate with clinical disease activity but did predict the group of patients who responded to lymphocytapheresis treatment[53], and has also been reported to be associated with characteristic cellular synovial membrane histology[54]. Although this system would not be suitable for regular disease assessment, it does suggest that monitoring cell-mediated immune activity may contribute important information about the complex immunological activity of rheumatoid arthritis.

Farr and colleagues measured serum and synovial fluid levels of adenosine deaminase, an enzyme associated with T-lymphocyte activity[55]. A rare deficiency of this enzyme[56] results in depressed cell-mediated immune responses. Adenosine deaminase levels increase significantly in the supernatants of phytohemagglutinin-stimulated lymphocytes. Farr and colleagues measured adenosine deaminase levels in the sera and synovial fluids of 28 rheumatoid arthritis patients, 11 osteoarthritis patients and 11 patients with other inflammatory arthropathies[55]. They found that serum adenosine deaminase levels were not significantly elevated in the inflammatory arthropathies. However, synovial fluid adenosine deaminase levels were significantly elevated in 93% of rheumatoid arthritis patients, 75% of the other arthropathies and 18% of osteoarthritis patients. There was a highly significant difference between the enzyme activity in rheumatoid arthritis and osteoarthritis synovial fluids. Adenosine deaminase levels correlated weakly with synovial fluid lymphocyte counts ($r = 0.349$) and orosomucoid levels ($r = 0.424$).

More recently, the expression of major histocompatibility complex class II antigens and the interleukin 2 receptor on peripheral blood T cells and the measurement of the serum concentration of soluble interleukin 2 receptor have been proposed as indices of cell-mediated immunity.

Measures of activated T lymphocytes in peripheral blood

Peripheral blood T-lymphocyte major histocompatibility complex class II expression

In the early 1980s there were several reports of elevated numbers of peripheral blood T lymphocytes expressing major histocompatibility complex class II antigens on their surface in rheumatoid arthritis[57-59]. However, a recent report suggested that such an increase was related to the presence of the genetic determinant B8 rather than to active inflammatory disease[60]. The only study using flow cytometric analysis found elevated numbers of class II positive peripheral blood T lymphocytes only in rheumatoid arthritis patients who had depressed *in vivo* lymphocyte responses to soluble antigens, regardless of clinical disease activity[54]. We studied 23 patients with rheumatoid arthritis and 22 age-matched controls for peripheral blood T-lymphocyte major histocompatibility complex class II (DR) expression in terms of the percentages of positive T lymphocytes and the intensity of fluorescence of T-lymphocyte DR expression[61]. We found that there was a large range of values in both the rheumatoid arthritis and control groups with no significant difference between them. There was also no correlation of T-lymphocyte DR expression and clinical disease activity.

Peripheral blood T-lymphocyte interleukin 2 receptor expression

Low levels of peripheral blood T-lymphocyte interleukin 2 receptor expression are found in both normal and rheumatoid subjects. Emery and colleagues studied 27 rheumatoid arthritis patients and 15 controls by flow cytometry[62]. They found that there was a significant increase in the percentage of T lymphocytes expressing the interleukin 2 receptor identified by the anti-TAC monoclonal antibody, in patients with active disease. Patients with inactive disease showed no difference from healthy controls.

Soluble interleukin 2 receptor

Interleukin 2 (IL-2) is a 15 kDa MW polypeptide that functions as a growth factor for T and B lymphocytes[63] and may play a role in the activation of monocytes[64]. Interleukin 2 acts via specific receptors on the cell surface. Expression of these interleukin 2 receptors on the cell surface increases after activation of peripheral blood mononuclear cells by mitogens, antigens and cytokines including interferon γ, interleukin 1 and interleukin 2 itself[65]. Two surface antigens together form the high affinity interleukin 2 receptor which is the receptor that enables cells to proliferate in response to interleukin 2[66]. One of these antigens is the low affinity interleukin 2 receptor of MW 55 kDa (the p55 subunit or α chain) which binds the anti-TAC monoclonal antibody[65]. The other antigen is a 75 kDa polypeptide with intermediate interleukin 2 binding affinity (the p70 subunit or β chain)[67]. Interleukin 2 promotes the rapid internalization of high affinity interleukin 2 receptor[68]. Internalization of the bound high affinity receptor is required for the signal transduction to stimulate proliferation. Low affinity interleukin 2 receptor does bind interleukin 2 but is not internalized and does not mediate proliferation. Membrane interleukin 2 receptor expression increases after activation of T lymphocytes and reaches a maximum within 2 days and then declines[69]. Corresponding to this decline is the finding of a 45 kDa interleukin 2 receptor (8–10 kDa lighter than the membrane low affinity interleukin 2 receptor) in the culture supernatant which reaches a maximum at 72 hours. This is called the soluble interleukin 2 receptor and is shed or secreted by stimulated T and B lymphocytes[70]. It has been demonstrated that soluble interleukin 2 receptor binds interleukin 2, with a similar affinity to the low affinity receptor in man[71]. The interleukin 2 receptor peptide has been demonstrated to end before its normal transmembrane and intracytoplasmic segments, at or before the amino acid Cys-192 of the full length molecule[72]. These investigators found no modification of the amino acid sequence of the soluble portion and concluded that the change was due to proteolysis which released the soluble interleukin 2 receptor rather than alternate mRNA splicing.

Using two monoclonal antibodies directed against non-overlapping epitopes on the interleukin 2 receptor, Rubin and colleagues[70] developed a 'sandwich' enzyme-linked immunosorbent assay (ELISA) for the quantitative measurement of soluble interleukin 2 receptor. The monoclonal antibodies used were anti-Tac and 7G7/B6. This system has been used to detect soluble interleukin 2 receptor in several immune-mediated diseases including leprosy patients during reversal reactions[73], rheumatoid arthritis[74] and liver transplant rejection[75]. Campen and colleagues measured soluble interleukin 2 receptor levels in 12 patients with rheumatoid arthritis and found a better correlation with disease activity (assessed by a joint index of the sum of scores 1–3 for each of 68 joints), than the erythrocyte sedimentation rate[76]. They also measured peripheral blood soluble interleukin 2 receptor levels in 26 systemic lupus erythematosus patients and found a good correlation with disease activity and complement levels. Soluble interleukin 2 receptor levels were also elevated in nine patients with subacute bacterial endocarditis but were not two standard deviations greater than normal mean values in ten patients with acute gout.

Higher levels of soluble interleukin 2 receptors are found in synovial fluid than in peripheral blood in rheumatoid arthritis patients suggesting that the synovial compartment is at least one site of production of soluble interleukin 2 receptors in rheumatoid arthritis. In systemic lupus erythematosus the sites of production are unknown. Unstimulated peripheral blood mononuclear cells from patients with systemic lupus erythematosus cultured *in vitro* release minimal amounts of soluble interleukin 2 receptors into the culture supernatant, suggesting an extravascular site of soluble interleukin 2 receptor production.

As the soluble interleukin 2 receptor binds interleukin 2, it has been suggested that it may represent a negative feedback pathway for immune system activation. An interleukin 2 inhibitor has been isolated from the synovial fluid of rheumatoid arthritis patients[77]. Symons and colleagues have suggested that the soluble interleukin 2 receptor may be this inhibitor[78]. There is a discrepancy in the size of the proteins with this activity which are approximately 90–100 kDa MW. Symons and colleagues have suggested that synovial fluid soluble interleukin 2 receptor proteins may occur as dimers which would have the appropriate molecular weight.

Regardless of the potential role that the soluble interleukin 2 receptor has in modulating immune responses, the facts that levels are raised in the peripheral blood of patients with rheumatoid arthritis and do fluctuate with changes in disease activity, suggest that soluble interleukin 2 receptor levels may provide a convenient way of monitoring immune activity in rheumatoid arthritis. However, much larger prospective studies are needed before the usefulness of this measure can be judged.

Plasma interleukin 1 levels

It has been known for several years that interleukin 1 is present in the synovial fluid of rheumatoid arthritis patients[79]. The presence of elevated levels of interleukin 1β has been detected in the peripheral blood of a group of rheumatoid arthritis patients by Eastgate and colleagues[80]. They found that levels of interleukin 1β correlated with a log scale of the Ritchie articular index and with erythrocyte sedimentation rate values. However, when a small number of patients were investigated longitudinally, the correlation with clinical and laboratory disease activity was not as strong. We have recently found that there is a significant reduction in the synovial membrane staining for interleukin 1β after the treatment of rheumatoid arthritis patients with gold. Although these tests change with changes in disease activity, their main role at present will be in elucidating important pathways of immune activation in rheumatoid arthritis. However, these findings allow an insight into how future rheumatologists may assess and categorize inflammatory arthropathies.

SUMMARY AND IMPLICATIONS

A large number of laboratory indicators of disease activity in rheumatoid arthritis have been and will continue to be proposed. In the past, many different indices have measured changes similar to those measured by the clinically well-characterized and researched erythrocyte sedimentation rate and C-reactive protein, and have thus not found a useful role. There are several indices which measure other aspects of rheumatoid arthritis disease activity, such as soluble interleukin 2 receptor, cartilage degradation products, neutrophil activation markers and the complement component C1q, which may find a useful role in providing *additional* information to the erythrocyte sedimentation rate or C-reactive protein. An example of a potentially important indicator of disease activity is the recent report by Stewart and colleagues[81] which described a technique for analyzing soluble collagen Type II (found only in hyaline cartilage) fragments in serum samples. This finding has the potential use for monitoring cartilage degradation in the arthropathies. New findings about the pathological processes involved in rheumatoid arthritis will also suggest new tests. For example, we have recently found that, although synovial membrane T-lymphocyte numbers do not change significantly in the first 3 months of gold and methylprednisolone therapy, there is a significant decline in endothelial cell expression of the neutrophil adhesion molecule, ELAM 1. This area of cellular adhesion molecules provides a good example of a rapidly expanding field that may produce important measures for assessing changes in disease activity.

These recent studies can thus provide insights into the modes of action of disease remitting agents and may also be useful ways of monitoring changes in disease activity. Prognostic indicators are also needed to indicate which patients require disease suppressing treatment before irreversible damage is done. This last point is at present of theoretical interest as there are no successful disease remitting agents currently in use, but those patients with poor prognostic indicators need to be identified for studies of the large numbers of proposed disease modifying agents awaiting trial.

There is, however, a major issue which must be addressed if the value of existing and experimental indicators of disease activity is to be assessed. Any study of laboratory indicators of disease activity must have a meaningful measure of disease outcome with which it can be compared. This could be, for example, joint erosion scores, disease activity as assessed clinically, or functional assessments such as that estimated by the Health Activity Questionnaire method, or any combination of these. If this issue can be resolved then large long-term collaborative studies can be organized. These studies are urgently required in order to establish the validity of competing claims in large enough numbers of patients followed for adequate periods of time. Perhaps the forum of an International Congress of Rheumatology is the most appropriate place for the initiation of such collaborative work.

ACKNOWLEDGEMENTS

Submitted in part for the MD degree of the University of Otago, New Zealand. Dr B. Kirkham was supported by the Dorothy Eden Fellowship, Arthritis Foundation of New Zealand Inc.

REFERENCES

1. Reizenstein, P. (1979). The haematological stress syndrome. *Br. J. Haematol.*, **43**, 329−34

2. Kushner, I. (1989). Erythrocyte sedimentation rate and the acute phase reactants. In Kelly, W.N., Harris, E.D., Ruddy, S. and Sledge, C.B. (eds.) *Textbook of Rheumatology*, 3rd edn., pp. 719−27. (Philadelphia: W.B. Saunders)

3. Pollack, W. (1965). Some physicochemical aspects of hemagglutination. *Ann. N.Y. Acad. Sci.*, **127**, 892−8

4. Talstad, I. and Haugen, H.F. (1979). The relationship between the erythrocyte sedimentation rate (ESR) and plasma proteins in clinical materials and models. *Scand. J. Clin. Lab. Invest.*, **39**, 519−24

5. Lascari, A.D. (1972). The erythrocyte sedimentation rate. *Pediatr. Clin. North. Am.*, **19**, 1113−21

6. Hutchinson, R.M. and Eastham, R.D. (1977). A comparison of the erythrocyte sedimentation rate and plasma viscosity in detecting changes in plasma proteins. *J. Clin. Pathol.*, **30**, 345−9

7. McCarty, M. (1982). Historical perspective on C-reactive protein. *Ann. N.Y. Acad. Sci.*, **389**, 1−10

8. Osmand, A.P., Friedenson, B., Gerwurz, H., Painter, R.H., Hoffman, T. and Shelton, E. (1977). Characterization of C-reactive protein and the complement subcomponent Clt as homologous proteins displaying cyclic pentameric symmetry (pentraxins). *Proc. Natl. Acad. Sci. USA*, **74**, 739−43

9. Kushner, I., Broder, M.L. and Karp, D. (1978). Control of the acute phase response: C-reactive protein kinetics after acute myocardial infarction. *J. Clin. Invest.*, **61**, 235−42

10. Morley, J.J. and Kushner, I. (1982). Serum C-reactive protein levels in disease. *Ann. N.Y. Acad. Sci.*, **389**, 406−18

11. Gushaw, J.B., Briscoe, R., Eimstad, W.M., Chang, C., Greenwood, H.M. and Allen, J.D. (1982). A simple, rapid enzyme immunoassay for C-reactive protein. *Ann. N.Y. Acad. Sci.*, **389**, 442−8

12. Glibetic, M.D. and Baumann, H. (1986). Influence of chronic inflammation

on the level of mRNA for acute-phase reactants in the mouse liver. *J. Immunol.*, **137**, 1616–22

13. Andus, T., Geiger, T., Hirano, T., Kishmoto, T. and Heinrich, P.C. (1988). Action of recombinant human interleukin 6, interleukin 1β and tumor necrosis factor α on the mRNA induction of acute-phase proteins. *Eur. J. Immunol.*, **18**, 739–46

14. Mortensen, R.F., Shapiro, J., Lin, B.-F., Douches, S. and Neta, R. (1988). Interaction of recombinant IL-1 and recombinant tumor necrosis factor in the induction of mouse acute phase proteins. *J. Immunol.*, **140**, 2260–6

15. Baumann, H., Richards, C. and Gauldie, J. (1987). Interaction among hepatocyte-stimulating factors, interleukin 1, and glucocorticoids for regulation of acute phase plasma proteins in human hepatoma (HepG2) cells. *J. Immunol.*, **139**, 4122–8

16. Dixon, J.S. (1984). Relationship between plasma viscosity or ESR and the Ritchie articular index (Letter). *Br. J. Rheumatol.*, **23**, 233–5

17. Pickup, M.E., Dixon, J.S., Hallet, C., Bird, H.A. and Wright, V. (1981). Plasma viscosity – a new appraisal of its use as an index of disease activity in rheumatoid arthritis. *Ann. Rheum. Dis.*, **40**, 272–5

18. Kelly, C.A., McClelland, J., Fail, B. and Walker, D. (1987). Erythrocyte sedimentation rate, plasma and serum viscosity as measures of disease activity in rheumatoid arthritis. *Br. J. Rheumatol.*, **26**, 136–8

19. Dixon, J.S. (1982). Biochemical and clinical changes in rheumatoid arthritis: their relation to the action of antirheumatoid drugs. *Sem. Arthr. Rheum.*, **12**, 191–207

20. Duthie, J.J.R., Brown, P.E., Truelove, L.H., Baragar, F.D. and Lawrie, A.J. (1964). Course and prognosis in rheumatoid arthritis. A further report. *Ann. Rheum. Dis.*, **23**, 193–202

21. Sherrer, Y.S., Bloch, D.A., Mitchell, D.M., Young, D.Y. and Fries, J.F. (1986). The development of disability in rheumatoid arthritis. *Arthr. Rheum.*, **26**, 494–500

22. Feigenbaum, S.L., Masi, A.T. and Kaplan, S.B. (1979). Prognosis in rheumatoid arthritis. A longitudinal study of newly diagnosed younger adult patients. *Am. J. Med.*, **66**, 377–84

23. Jacoby, R.K., Jayson, M.I.V. and Cosh, J.A. (1973). Onset, early stages and prognosis of rheumatoid arthritis: a clinical study of 100 patients with 11 year follow-up. *Br. Med. J.*, **2**, 96–100

24. Scott, D.L., Dawes, P.T., Fowler, P.D., Grindulis, K.A., Shadforth, M. and Bacon, P.A. (1985). Anti-rheumatic drugs and joint damage in rheumatoid arthritis. *Q. J. Med.*, **54**, 49–59

25. Sjoblom, K.G., Saxne, T., Pettersson, H. and Wollheim, F.A. (1984).

Factors related to the progression of joint destruction in rheumatoid arthritis. *Scand. J. Rheumatol.*, **13**, 21–7

26. Amos, R.S., Constable, T.J., Crockson, A.P. and McConkey, B. (1977). Rheumatoid arthritis: relation of serum C-reactive protein and erythrocyte sedimentation rates to radiographic changes. *Br. Med. J.*, **1**, 195–7

27. Dawes, P.T., Fowler, P.D., Jackson, R., Collins, M., Shadforth, M.F., Stone, R. and Scott, D.L. (1986). Prediction of progressive joint damage in patients with rheumatoid arthritis receiving gold or D-penicillamine therapy. *Ann. Rheum. Dis.*, **45**, 945–9

28. Gorevic, P.D., Rosenthal, C.J. and Franklin, E.C. (1976). Amyloid-related serum component (SAA) – studies in acute infections, medullary thyroid carcinoma, and post surgery. *Clin. Immunol. Immunopathol.*, **6**, 83–93

29. Chambers, R.E., Macfarlane, D.G., Whicher, J.T. and Dieppe, P.A. (1983). Serum amyloid-A protein concentration in rheumatoid arthritis and its role in monitoring disease activity. *Ann. Rheum. Dis.*, **42**, 665–7

30. Grindulis, K.A., Scott, D.L., Robinson, M.W., Bacon, P.A. and McConkey, B. (1985). Serum amyloid A protein during the treatment of rheumatoid arthritis with second-line drugs. *Br. J. Rheumatol.*, **24**, 158–63

31. Surrall, K.E., Bird, H.A. and Dixon, J.S. (1987). Caeruloplasmin, prealbumin and α_2-macroglobulin as potential indices of disease activity in different arthritides. *Clin. Rheumatol.*, **6**, 64–9

32. Dawes, P.T., Jackson, R., Shadforth, M.F., Lewin, I.V. and Stanworth, D.R. (1987). The relationship between the complex of immunoglobulin A and alpha-1-antitrypsin, its constituent components and the acute-phase response as measured by C-reactive protein in rheumatoid arthritis treated with gold or D-penicillamine. *Br. J. Rheumatol.*, **26**, 351–3

33. Gerber, D.A. (1975). Low free serum histidine concentration in rheumatoid arthritis – a measure of disease activity. *J. Clin. Invest.*, **55**, 1164–73

34. Pickup, M.E., Dixon, J.S., Lowe, J.R. and Wright, V. (1980). Serum histidine in rheumatoid arthritis: changes induced by anti-rheumatic drug therapy. *J. Rheumatol.*, **7**, 71–6

35. Gerber, D.A. and Gerber, M.G. (1977). Specificity of a low free serum histidine concentration for rheumatoid arthritis. *J. Chron. Dis.*, **30**, 115–27

36. Sitton, N.G., Dixon, J.S., Bird, H.A. and Wright, V. (1987). Serum biochemistry in rheumatoid arthritis, seronegative arthropathies, osteoarthritis, SLE and normal subjects. *Br. J. Rheumatol.*, **26**, 131–5

37. Lorber, A., Bovy, R.A. and Chang, C.C. (1971). Sulphydryl deficiency in connective tissue disorders: correlation with disease activity and protein alterations. *Metabolism*, **20**, 446–55

38. Pickup, M.E., Dixon, J.S. and Bird, H.A. (1980). On the effects of anti-rheumatic drugs on protein sulphydryl reactivity in human serum. *J. Pharm. Pharmacol.*, **32**, 301–2

39. Woolfe, A.D., Hall, N.D., Kanthria, B., Maymo, J., Goulding, N.J. and Maddison, P.J. (1986). Predictors of 5 year outcome of early synovitis (Abstract). *Br. J. Rheumatol.*, **25** (Suppl. 2), 23–4

40. Thompson, P.W., Jones, D.D. and Currey, H.L.F. (1986). Cytidine deaminase activity as a measure of acute inflammation in rheumatoid arthritis. *Ann. Rheum. Dis.*, **45**, 9–14

41. Thompson, P.W., Kirwin, J.R., Jones, D.D. and Currey, H.L.F. (1986). Serial blood levels of cytidine deaminase can detect the flare produced by the withdrawal of non-steroidal anti-inflammatory therapy in RA patients. *Br. J. Rheumatol.*, **25** (Suppl. 2), 79

42. Adeyemi, E.O., Hull, R.G., Chadwick, V.S., Hughes, G.R.V. and Hodgson, H.J.F. (1986). Circulating human leukocyte elastase in rheumatoid arthritis. *Rheumatol. Int.*, **6**, 57–60

43. Saxne, T., Heinegard, D. and Wollheim, F.A. (1986). Therapeutic effects on cartilage metabolism in arthritis as measured by release of proteoglycan structures into the synovial fluid. *Ann. Rheum. Dis.*, **45**, 419–7

44. Saxne, T., Wollheim, F.A., Petterson, H. and Heinegard, D. (1987). Proteoglycan concentration in synovial fluid: predictor of future cartilage destruction in rheumatoid arthritis? *Br. Med. J.*, **295**, 1447–8

45. Chuck, A.J., Murphy, J., Weiss, J.B. and Greenan, D.M. (1986). Comparison of urinary glycosaminoglycan excretion in rheumatoid arthritis, osteoarthritis, myocardial infarction and controls. *Ann. Rheum. Dis.*, **45**, 162–6

46. Ochi, T., Yonemasu, K., Iwase, R., Sasaki, T., Tsuyama, K. and Ono, K. (1984). Serum C1q levels as a prognostic guide to articular erosions in patients with rheumatoid arthritis. *Arthr. Rheum.*, **27**, 883–7

47. Ochi, T., Iwase, R., Yonemasu, K., Matsukawa, M., Yoneda, M., Yukioka, M. and Ono, K. (1988). Natural course of joint destruction and fluctuation of serum C1q levels in patients with rheumatoid arthritis. *Arthr. Rheum.*, **31**, 37–43

48. Mottonen, T., Hannonen, P., Rautianen, J., Jokinen, I., Oka, M. and Arvilommi, H. (1989). Serum C1q level does not predict joint erosion in early rheumatoid arthritis. *Arthr. Rheum.*, **32**, 511–12

49. Bull, B.S., Levy, W.C., Westengard, J.C., Farr, M., Smith, P.F., Apperly, J.F., Bacon, P.A. and Stuart, J. (1986). Ranking of laboratory tests by consensus analysis. *Lancet*, **2**, 377–80

50. Paulus, H.E., Machleder, H.I., Levine, S., Yu, D.T.Y. and Macdonald, N.S. (1977). Lymphocyte involvement in rheumatoid arthritis. Studies

during thoracic duct drainage. *Arthr. Rheum.*, **20**, 1249–62

51. Janossy, G., Panayi, G.S., Duke, O., Bofill, M., Poulter, L.W. and Goldstein, G. (1981). Rheumatoid arthritis: a disease of T lymphocyte/macrophage immunoregulation. *Lancet*, **2**, 839–42

52. Emery, P., Panayi, G.S. and Nouri, A.M.E. (1984). Interleukin-2 reverses deficient cell-mediated immune responses in rheumatoid arthritis. *Clin. Exp. Immunol.*, **57**, 123–9

53. Wahl, S.M., Wilder, R.L., Katona, I.L., Wahl, L.M., Allen, J.B., Scher, I. and Decker, J.L. (1983). Leukapheresis in rheumatoid arthritis: association of clinical improvement with reversal of anergy. *Arthr. Rheum.*, **26**, 1076–84

54. Haraoui, B., Wilder, R.L., Malone, D.G., Allen, J.B., Katona, I.M. and Wahl, S.M. (1984). Immune function in severe, active rheumatoid arthritis: a relationship between peripheral blood mononuclear cell proliferation to soluble antigens and mononuclear cell subset profiles. *J. Immunol.*, **133**, 697–701

55. Farr, M., Buckley, B., Smedley, S. and Bacon, P.A. (1987). Adenosine deaminase (ADA) in synovial fluid: a new measure for local joint inflammation? *Br. J. Rheumatol.*, **26** (Abstr. Suppl. 1), 2–3

56. Thompson, L.F. and Seegmiller, J.E. (1980). Adenosine deaminase deficiency and severe combined immunodeficiency disease. *Adv. Enzymol.*, **58**, 167–210

57. Burmester, G.R., Jahn, B., Gramatziki, M., Zacher, J. and Kalden, J.R. (1984). Activated T cells *in vivo* and *in vitro*: divergence in expression of Tac and Ia antigens in the nonblastoid small T cells of inflammation and normal T cells activated *in vitro*. *J. Immunol.*, **133**, 1230–4

58. Fox, R.I., Fong, S., Sabharwal, N., Carstens, S.A., Kung, P.C. and Vaughan, J.H. (1982). Synovial fluid lymphocytes differ from peripheral blood lymphocytes in patients with rheumatoid arthritis. *J. Immunol.*, **128**, 351–4

59. Pincus, S.H., Clegg, D.O. and Ward, J.R. (1985). Characterization of T cells bearing HLA-DR antigens in rheumatoid arthritis. *Arthr. Rheum.*, **28**, 8–15

60. Clegg, D.O., Pincus, S.H., Zone, J.J. and Ward, J.R. (1986). Circulating HLA-DR bearing T cells: correlation with genetic rather than clinical variables. *J. Rheumatol.*, **13**, 870–4

61. Kirkham, B.W., Pitzalis, C., Kingsley, G.H., Timms, A.M., Kyriazis, N. and Panayi, G.S. (1989). Rheumatoid T lymphocyte MHC Class II expression: *in vitro* stimulation produces normal MHC Class II proliferation, independent of proliferation. *J. Rheumatol.*, **14**, 270–5

62. Emery, P., Wood, N., Gentry, K., Stockman, A., Mackay, I.R. and

Bernard, O. (1988). High-affinity interleukin-2 receptors on blood lymphocytes are decreased during active rheumatoid arthritis. *Arthr. Rheum.*, **31**, 1176–82

63. Mingari, M.C., Gerosa, F., Carra, G., Accolla, R.S., Moretta, A., Zubler, R.H., Waldmann, T.A. and Moretta, L. (1984). Human interleukin-2 promotes proliferation of activated B cells via surface receptors similar to those of activated T cells. *Nature (London)*, **312**, 641–3

64. Wahl, S.M., McCartney-Francis, N., Hunt, D.A., Smith, P.D., Wahl, L.M. and Katona, I.M. (1987). Monocyte interleukin-2 receptor gene expression and interleukin-2 augmentation of microbiocidal activity. *J. Immunol.*, **139**, 1342–7

65. Greene, W.C. and Leonard, W.J. (1986). The human interleukin-2 receptor. *Ann. Rev. Immunol.*, **4**, 69–95

66. Wang, H-M. and Smith, K.A. (1987). The interleukin-2 receptor: functional consequences of its bimolecular structure. *J. Exp. Med.*, **166**, 1055–64

67. Teshigawara, K., Wang, H-M., Kato, K. and Smith, K.A. (1987). Interleukin-2 high-affinity receptor expression requires two distinct binding proteins. *J. Exp. Med.*, **165**, 223–8

68. Fujii, M., Sugamura, K., Sano, K., Nakai, M., Sugita, K. and Hinuma, Y. (1986). High-affinity receptor-mediated internalization and degradation of interleukin-2 in human T cells. *J. Exp. Med.*, **163**, 550–62

69. Depper, J.M., Leonard, W.J., Kronke, M., Noguchi, P.D., Cunningham, R.E., Waldmann, T.A. and Greene, W.C. (1984). Regulation of interleukin-2 receptor expression: effects of phorbol diester, phospholipase C, and re-exposure to lectin or antigen. *J. Immunol.*, **133**, 3054–61

70. Rubin, L.A., Kurman, C.C., Fritz, M.E., Biddison, W.E., Boutin, B., Yarchoan, R. and Nelson, D.L. (1985). Soluble interleukin-2 receptors are released from activated human lymphoid cells *in vitro*. *J. Immunol.*, **135**, 3172–7

71. Jacques, Y., Le Mauff, B., Boeffard, F., Godard, A. and Soulillou, J-P. (1987). A soluble interleukin-2 receptor produced by a normal alloreactive human T cell clone binds interleukin-2 with low affinity. *J. Immunol.*, **139**, 2308–16

72. Robb, R.J. and Kutny, R.M. (1987). Structure–function relationships for the IL-2 receptor system. IV. Analysis of the sequence and ligand-binding properties of soluble Tac protein. *J. Immunol.*, **139**, 855–62

73. Tung, K.S.K., Umland, E., Matzner, P., Nelson, K., Schauf, V., Rubin, L., Wagner, D., Scollard, D., Vithayasai, P., Vithayasai, V., Worobic, S., Smith, T. and Surifanond, V. (1987). Soluble serum interleukin-2 receptor levels in leprosy patients. *Clin. Exp. Immunol.*, **69**, 10–15

74. Wood, N.C., Symons, J.A. and Duff, G.W. (1988). Serum interleukin-2-

receptor in rheumatoid arthritis: a prognostic indicator of disease activity? *J. Autoimmunity,* **1**, 353–61

75. Adams, D.H., Wang, L., Hubscher, S.G., Elias, E. and Neuberger, J.M. (1989). Soluble interleukin-2 receptors in serum and bile of liver transplant recipients. *Lancet,* **1**, 469–71

76. Campen, D.H., Horwitz, D.A., Quismorio, F.P., Ehresmann, G.R. and Martin, W.J. (1988). Serum levels of interleukin-2 receptor and activity of rheumatic diseases characterized by immune system activation. *Arthr. Rheum.,* **31**, 1358–64

77. Miossec, P., Kashiwado, T. and Ziff, M. (1987). Inhibitor of interleukin-2 in rheumatoid synovial fluid. *Arthr. Rheum.,* **30**, 121–9

78. Symons, J.A., Wood, N.C., Di Giovine, F.S. and Duff, G.W. (1988). Soluble IL-2 receptor in rheumatoid arthritis. Correlation with disease activity, IL-1 and IL-2 inhibition. *J. Immunol.,* **141**, 2612–18

79. Hopkins, S.J., Humphreys, M. and Jayson, M.I.V. (1988). Cytokines in synovial fluid. I. The presence of biologically active and immunoreactive IL-1. *Clin. Exp. Immunol.,* **72**, 422–7

80. Eastgate, J.A., Symons, J.A., Wood, N.C., Grinlinton, F.M., Di Giovine, F.S. and Duff, G.W. (1988). Correlation of plasma interleukin 1 levels with disease activity in rheumatoid arthritis. *Lancet,* **2**, 706–8

81. Stewart, T.E., Mestecky, J., Moreland, L.W. and Gay, S. (1989). Immunoassay for collagen type II (cII) in synovial fluid and serum of patients with erosive joint diseases. *Arthr. Rheum.,* **32**, S74

3

Modulation of bone metabolism by cyclosporin A

H. Skjødt, D.E. Hughes, T. Møller, D. AlFadl, A. AlHumidan and R.G.G. Russell

CYCLOSPORIN A AND CYTOKINE PRODUCTION

Cyclosporin A has proven to be a selective inhibitor of cytokines involved in the regulation of immune cell activation. Within the immune system, the activity spectrum of cyclosporin A appears to be restricted to lymphocytes. All sustained immune responses involve activation of T lymphocytes. Cyclosporin A inhibition of T-cell priming[1] is a key event in cyclosporin A immunosuppression. In particular, cyclosporin A inhibits *de novo* synthesis of interleukin 2[2], interleukin 3[3], interleukin 4[4] and interferon γ[5] as shown at the mRNA level in activated T cells (Figure 1). By contrast, synthesis of granulocyte macrophage colony stimulating factors in T cells appears to be cyclosporin A-resistant[3]. Cyclosporin A action is not restricted to T cells, however, as certain B-cell responses are cyclosporin A-sensitive (reviewed in ref. 6). No direct effect on interleukin 1 production by macrophages has been described, whereas tumor necrosis factor α production may be cyclosporin A-sensitive without affecting tumor necrosis factor mRNA levels[7]. The processing of antigen by antigen presenting cells (including monocytes, dendritic cells and B cells) appears to be unaffected by cyclosporin A[8] although controversy exists[9]. Nevertheless, induction of major histocompatibility complex class II determinants necessary for antigen presenting cell function is cyclosporin

43

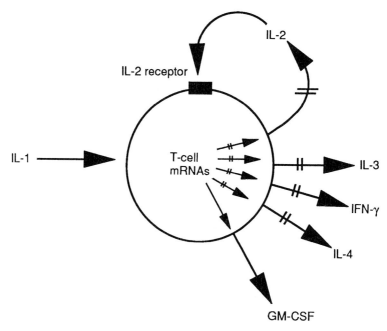

Figure 1 Cyclosporin A (CsA) is thought to act on T-helper cells (CD4+) by selectively inhibiting the transcription of mRNAs for cytokines, which include several interleukins (IL-2, IL-3, IL-4) and interferon γ (IFN-γ). The effects on IL-2 are particularly important in the immunosuppressive actions of cyclosporin A. GM-CSF = granulocyte macrophage stimulating factor

A-sensitive[10], probably through inhibition of interferon γ and interleukin 4 production by T cells. The complexity of the cytokine network, meaning that multiple cytokines are acting concurrently on cell types with distinct responses including cytokine- and cytokine receptor-production[11], suggests that cyclosporin A may act in a selective manner by inhibiting transcription of identical cytokines in different cell types. Also, many cytokines are not produced constitutively which may restrict cyclosporin A activity to certain phases of cell responsiveness.

IS CYCLOSPORIN A ACTION RESTRICTED TO THE IMMUNE SYSTEM?

Although surface receptors for cyclosporin A have been described[12], in general the lipophilic cyclosporin A molecule is thought to gain access to the cytoplasm of any cell type by simple diffusion across the membrane. Toxic effects described in hepatocytes and renal tubular and endothelial cells[13] may be distinguishable from the immunosuppressive properties of cyclosporin A. Cyclophilin is a cytoplasmic high-affinity cyclosporin A-binding protein and the binding of cyclosporins to such protein(s) appears to be closely linked to the immunosuppressive action of cyclosporins[14]. Recently, cyclophilin has been identified as the enzyme peptidyl-prolyl *cis-trans* isomerase[15,16]. By regulating protein folding during cell protein synthesis, peptidyl-prolyl *cis-trans* isomerase may play a pivotal role in defining the functional state of many cell proteins. Cyclosporin A blocks peptidyl-prolyl *cis-trans* isomerase activity[16] which may play a part in its selective inhibition of cytokine-gene transcription. Also, the ubiquitous presence of cyclophilins and peptidyl-prolyl *cis-trans* isomerase raises the question of whether cyclosporin A may inhibit cytokine production or otherwise alter protein synthesis in non-immune cells. Nonetheless, cyclosporin A inhibition of identical gene expression in different cells may still be highly dependent on the cell type[17].

THE SIGNIFICANCE OF CYTOKINE ACTIVITY IN A CONNECTIVE TISSUE: BONE

Although production of some cytokines, such as interleukin-2, appears restricted to the immune system, recent studies indicate that many cytokines – originally defined as immune cell mediators – are produced in a wide variety of non-immune cells (summarized in ref. 18). For example, bone has been the subject of much effort to clarify the possible role of a number of cytokines modulating bone cell activity *in vitro*. In particular, interleukin 1, tumor necrosis factor α and tumor necrosis factor β (lymphotoxin) are potent stimulators of bone resorption and also affect osteoblast metabolism. Interferon γ preferentially inhibits this cytokine-stimulated resorption. Further, colony stimulating factors including granulocyte macrophage colony stimulating factors are involved in the induction of osteoclasts in hemopoietic marrow (for a review of cytokines and bone, see ref. 19). In fact, bone cells may be a local source of many cytokines such as interleukin 1[20], tumor necrosis factor α (M. Gowen, personal communication) and colony stimulating factors[21] which are released during cell culture. The study of a putative local bone cytokine network awaits determination of cytokine mRNA expression in bone surface cells. In addition to bone stromal cells and osteoblasts, hemopoietic cells, osteoclasts and immune system cells are all present in the microenvironment of the bone remodeling surface.

Recently, we described expression of major histocompatibility complex class II determinants (HLA-DR and DQ) by a subset of human osteoblast-like bone surface cells in long-term culture[22]. Moreover, human bone cells stimulate proliferation of allogeneic and autologous peripheral blood mononuclear cells in co-culture and function as antigen presenting cells[23]. The major histocompatibility complex class II expression by human bone cells is enhanced by interferon γ and 1,25 dihydroxy vitamin D_3[22]. Activation of T cells including release of osteotropic cytokines could be involved in some regulatory pathways within bone.

ACTIVITY OF CYCLOSPORIN A ON BONE

The interactions between bone stromal cells and immune cells, including cytokine production, prompted studies on possible cyclosporin A modulation of bone cell metabolism. Thus, cyclosporin A inhibits the bone resorbing activity of interleukin 1, 1,25 dihydroxy vitamin D_3, parathyroid hormone and prostaglandin E_2 in two different bioassays of bone resorption[24-27] (Figure 2 and Table 1). This inhibitory effect is reversible, and appears independent of any significant cytotoxicity. Moreover, cyclosporin A has no apparent effect on basal calcium release from the organ cultures, nor on the endogenous induction of interleukin 1 by other cytokines. However, cyclosporin A antagonizes constitutive and interferon γ-stimulated HLA-DR expression by human bone cells, suggesting a possible inhibition of major histocompatibility complex class II stimulating factor(s) in the cultures (Skjødt, unpublished). In addition, interleukin 1-stimulated prostaglandin E_2 production in human bone cells as well as human articular chondrocyte cultures is inhibited by cyclosporin A[24]. The cyclosporin A inhibitory effect on the bone resorbing factors, however, is not mediated by inhibition of prostaglandin E_2, as revealed by addition of indomethacin (Skjødt, unpublished). Interestingly, the non-immunosuppressive analog, cyclosporin H, has no effect in the assays.

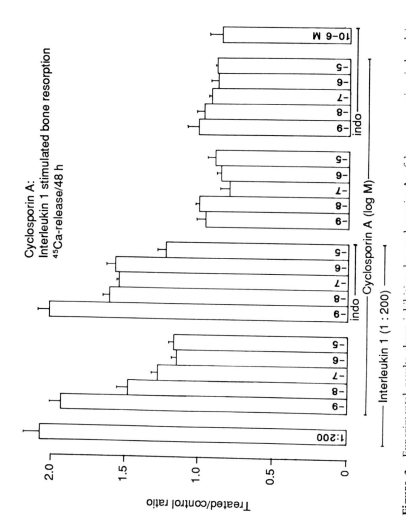

Figure 2 Experimental results show inhibition by cyclosporin A of bone resorption induced in mouse calvaria *in vitro*. In these experiments[24] interleukin 1β was used as the stimulator of bone resorption. Cyclosporin A also inhibits bone resorption induced by other agents[26,27]

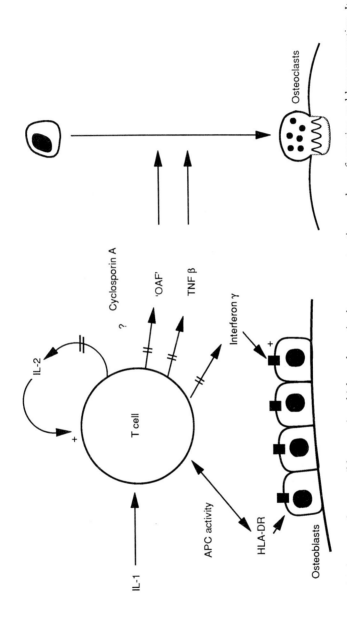

Figure 3 A scheme to show possible ways in which cyclosporin A may exert actions on bone formation and bone resorption. It is postulated that cyclosporin A acts principally by inhibiting the production of cytokines from T cells, which may be involved in mediating bone resorption and in enhancing (e.g. by induction of HLA class II antigens by interferon γ) the interaction between bone cells and T cells. It is also possible that cyclosporin A may have direct actions on bone cells to block production of bone-resorbing cytokines. TNF = tumor necrosis factor; APC = antigen presenting cell; IL = interleukin; OAF = osteoclast activating factors

Table 1 Summary of some properties of cyclosporin A which may be important in understanding its effects within bone

---

Cyclosporin A inhibits bone resorption *in vitro* when induced by several agents (e.g. interleukin 1, 1,25 dihyroxy vitamin D_3, prostaglandins)

Osteoblasts express HLA class II antigens, induced by interferon γ

Osteoblasts may act as antigen presenting cells

Are T cells in bone involved in cyclosporin A responses?

Are there non-T-cell effects of cyclosporin A?

In contrast, *in vivo* studies show conflicting results in terms of cyclosporin A inhibition of bone resorption and stimulation of bone formation[28] and, on the other hand, induction of severe bone resorption by cyclosporin A[29]. This may reflect the different dose regimes used and certainly stresses the point that any *in vivo* modulation by cyclosporin A of a complex cytokine network is not tested in the *in vitro* models used. In particular, target cells of cyclosporin A action in bone have not been identified: first, in the bone organ cultures T cells may be present, whereas second, in the human bone cell cultures no markers of immune cells (monocytes, T and B lymphocytes) have been found[22]. The question remains, however, whether cyclosporin A modulates stromal bone cells directly and/or acts through immunosuppressive effects in bone. The possible effects of cyclosporin A on T cells and bone are summarized in Figure 3. Further studies are needed on modulation of cytokine production by cyclosporin A in connective tissue cells.

ACKNOWLEDGEMENT

H. Skjødt is financially supported by The Danish Rheumatism Association (Gigtforeningen).

REFERENCES

1. Borel, J., Feurer, C., Magnee, C. and Stahelin, H. (1977). Effects of the new anti-lymphocytic peptide cyclosporin A in animals. *Immunology*, **32**, 1017–25

2. Kronke, M., Leonard, W.J., Depper, J.M., Arya, S.K., Wong-Staal, F., Gallo, R.C., Waldmann, T.A. and Greene, W.C. (1984). Cyclosporin A inhibits T-cell growth factor gene expression at the level of mRNA transcription. *Proc. Natl. Acad. Sci. USA,* **81,** 5214–18

3. Bickel, M., Tsuda, H., Amstad, P. *et al.* (1987). Differential regulation of colony-stimulating factors and interleukin 2 production by cyclosporin A. *Proc. Natl. Acad. Sci. USA,* **84,** 3274

4. Sideras, P., Funa, K., Zalcberg-Quintana, I., Xanthopoulos, K.G., Kieselow, P. and Palacios, R. (1988). Analysis by *in situ* hybridization of cells expressing mRNA for IL-4 in the developing thymus and in peripheral lymphocytes from mice. *Proc. Natl. Acad. Sci. USA,* **85,** 218

5. Reem, G.H., Cook, L.A. and Vilcek, J. (1983). Gamma interferon synthesis by human thymocytes and T lymphocytes inhibited by cyclosporin A. *Science,* **221,** 63–5

6. Klaus, G.G.B. (1988). Cyclosporine-sensitive and cyclosporine-insensitive modes of B cell stimulation. *Transplantation,* **46,** 11S–14S

7. Renneich, D.G., Nguyen, D.T., Eskandari, M.K., Strieter, R.M. and Kunkel, S.L. (1989). Cyclosporine A inhibits TNF production without decreasing TNF mRNA levels. *Biochem. Biophys. Res. Commun.,* **161,** 551–5

8. Muller, S., Adorini, L., Appella, E. and Nagy, Z.A. (1988). Lack of influence of cyclosporine on antigen presentation to lysozyme-specific T cell hybridomas. *Transplantation,* **46,** 44S–48S

9. Palay, D.A., Cluff, C.W., Wentworth, P.A. and Ziegler, H.K. (1986). Cyclosporine inhibits macrophage-mediated antigen presentation. *J. Immunol.,* **136,** 4348–53

10. Buurman, W.A., Groenewegen, G., van der Linden, C.J. and Kootstra, C. (1986). MHC class II expression and cyclosporin. *Transplant Proc.,* **18,** 855–6

11. Balkwill, F.R. and Burke, F. (1989). The cytokine network. *Immunol. Today,* **10,** 299–304

12. Ryffel, B., Donatsch, P., Gotz, U. and Tschopp, M. (1980). Cyclosporin receptor on mouse lymphocytes. *Immunology,* **41,** 913–19

13. Ziegler, K., Frimmer, M. and Koepsell, H. (1988). Photoaffinity labeling of membrane proteins from rat liver and pig kidney with cyclosporine diazirine. *Transplantation,* **46,** 15S–20S

14. Handschumacher, R.E., Harding, M.W., Rice, J., Drugge, R.J. and Speicher, D.W. (1984). Cyclophilin: a specific cytosolic binding protein for cyclosporin A. *Science,* **226,** 544–7

15. Fischer, G., Wittmann-Liebold, B., Lang, K., Kiefhaber, T. and Schmid, F.X. (1989). Cyclophilin and peptidyl-prolyl *cis-trans* isomerase are probably identical proteins. *Nature (London),* **337,** 476–8

16. Takahashi, N., Hayano, T. and Suzuki, M. (1989). Peptidyl-prolyl *cis-trans* isomerase is the cyclosporin A-binding protein cyclophilin. *Nature (London)*, **337**, 473–5

17. Gunter, K.C., Irving, S.G., Zipfel, P.F., Siebenlist, U. and Kelly, K. (1989). Cyclosporin A-mediated inhibition of mitogen-induced gene transcription is specific for the mitogenic stimulus and cell type. *J. Immunol.*, **142**, 3286–91

18. Green, A.R. (1989). Peptide regulatory factors: multifunctional mediators of cellular growth and differentiation. *Lancet*, **1**, 705-7

19. Gowen, M. (1988). The relationship between the immune system and bone formation and destruction. *Bone. Clin. Biochem. News Rev.*, **5**, 34–6

20. Hughes, D.E., Gowen, M. and Russell, R.G.G. (1988). Interleukin 1 as a paracrine factor in bone: effects on osteoclast-like cell formation and production by osteoblast-like cells. *J. Bone Min. Res.*, **3**, S196 (abstr.)

21. Elford, P.R., Felix, R., Cecchini, M., Trechsel, U. and Fleisch, H. (1986). Murine osteoblast-like cells and the osteogenic cell MC3T3-E1 release a macrophage colony stimulating activity in culture. *Calc. Tiss. Int.*, **41**, 151–7

22. Skjødt, H., Hughes, D.E., Dobson, P.R.M. and Russell, R.G.G. (1989). Constitutive and inducible expression of HLA class II determinants by human osteoblast-like cells *in vitro*. *J. Clin. Invest.*, in press

23. Skjødt, H., Møller, T. and Freiesleben, S. (1989). Human osteoblast-like cells expressing MHC class II determinants stimulate allogeneic and autologous peripheral blood mononuclear cells and function as antigen presenting cells. *Immunology*, in press

24. Skjødt, H., Crawford, A., Elford, P.R., Ihrie, E., Wood, D.D. and Russell, R.G.G. (1985). Cyclosporin A modulates interleukin-1 activity on bone *in vitro*. *Br. J. Rheumatol.*, **24**, 165–9

25. Skjødt, H., Beresford, J.N., Wood, D.D. and Russell, R.G.G. (1985). Interleukin 1 and cyclosporin A modulate actions of 1,25-dihydroxyvitamin D_3 on bone *in vitro*. In Norman, A.W. *et al.* (eds.) *Vitamin D: Chemical, Biochemical and Clinical Update*, pp. 491–2. (Berlin: W. de Gruyter)

26. Stewart, P.J., Green, O.C. and Stern, P.H. (1986). Cyclosporine A inhibits calcemic hormone-induced bone resorption *in vitro*. *J. Bone Min. Res.*, **1**, 285–91

27. Klaushofer, K., Hoffmann, O., Stewart, P.J., Czerwenka, E., Koller, K., Peterlik, M. and Stern, P.H. (1987). Cyclosporine A inhibits bone resorption in cultured neonatal mouse calvaria. *J. Pharm. Exp. Ther.*, **243**, 584–90

28. Orcel, P., Bielakoff, J., Modrowski, D., Miravet, L. and Vernejoul, M.C. (1989). Cyclosporin A induces *in vivo* inhibition of resorption and

stimulation of formation in rat bone. *J. Bone Min. Res.,* **4**, 387-91

29. Movsowitz, C., Epstein, S., Fallon, M., Ismail, F. and Thomas, S. (1988). Cyclosporin-A *in vivo* produces severe osteopenia in the rat: effect of dose and duration of administration. *Endocrinology,* **123**, 2571-7

4

Effect of Sandimmun® on bone remodeling in normal rats and under various pathological conditions

E. del Pozo, P. Elford, J.P Casez, J. Gale, M. Graeber and T. Payne

INTRODUCTION

Cyclosporin A (Sandimmun®) is a metabolite of the soil fungi *Tolypocladium inflatum gams*, and is widely used in the prevention of rejection following solid organ transplantation procedures. Sandimmun® exerts its immunosuppressive effect by selectively inhibiting the transcription of mRNA for interleukin 2 and other lymphokines in T lymphocytes[1]. Since interleukin 2 is required for the activation of T-helper cells and cytolytic T cells, Sandimmun® might be expected to act in adjuvant arthritis by inhibiting interleukin 2 production. However, evidence has been recently provided for a direct effect of Sandimmun® on interleukin 1, a cytokine implicated in the control of bone and calcium turnover[2]. Although the spectrum of actions of this compound has been widely investigated in the laboratory animal and in man[3], results of studies on bone remodeling have been controversial. Thus, Sandimmun® has been found to counteract *in vitro* release of calcium induced by parathyroid hormone, vitamin D1-25 and osteoclast-activating factor, whereas the compound alone had no effect[4], and evidence has been recently provided for a mechanism of action via suppression of immunological phenomena[5]. More recently, Orcel and colleagues[6] have recorded *in vivo* suppression of bone resorption by Sandimmun® in untreated rats. They also observed enhanced bone apposition in vertebrae as estimated by dynamic histomorphometry after double tetracycline labeling. However, these results are at variance with recent publications showing tibial osteopenia and osteocalcin elevation subsequent to Sandimmun® administration to normal rats[7] with partial recovery on discontinuation of treatment[8].

The current studies report the effects of Sandimmun® on interleukin 1-induced bone resorption *in vitro* as well as its effects on bone metabolism in normal rats, rats with adjuvant arthritis and in animals with a renal allograft.

EFFECT OF SANDIMMUN® ON INTERLEUKIN 1-INDUCED BONE RESORPTION *IN VITRO*

Calvaria dissected from 6-day-old CD-1 mice were bisected and cultured for 4 days in Bigger's medium (BGJ) with 0.1% low-endotoxin bovine serum albumin, in the presence of recombinant human interleukin 1β (a gift from Dr Tagliabue, Sclavo Research Center, Sienna, Italy), with or without Sandimmun®. The calcium concentration of the culture medium was then determined spectrophotometrically ('Ca-Kit', Bio-Mérieux, Charbonnières les Bains, France). Calvaria were embedded in methyl-methacrylate and 5 μm sections stained for tartrate-resistant acid phosphatase, in order to enumerate osteoclasts. The cross-sectional area of calvarial sections was determined using a computer-assisted imaging analyzer (Imaging Inc., Brock University, Ontario, Canada).

Sandimmun® reduced interleukin 1-induced bone resorption in a concentration-dependent manner (Figure 1). This was mirrored by an inhibition in the rise of osteoclast numbers induced by interleukin 1 (Figure 2), implying that Sandimmun® blocks bone resorption not by an effect upon pre-existing osteoclasts, but by preventing osteoclastic recruitment. Our results confirm and extend those of others using the same calvarial bone resorption system[9,10]. However, since we observed a large release of lactate dehydrogenase (indicating cellular toxicity) at a concentration of compound only twice (8 μmol/l) that causing complete inhibition of bone resorption, it cannot be excluded that at least part of the inhibitory property of Sandimmun® in this *in vitro* system could be due to toxicity.

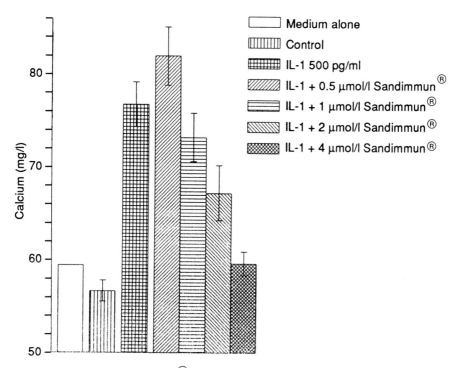

Figure 1   Effect of Sandimmun® on interleukin 1 (IL-1)-induced release of calcium in medium of calvarial cultures. There is a clear dose-dependent inhibition

SKELETAL RESPONSE TO CHRONIC ADMINIS-
TRATION OF SANDIMMUN® TO NORMAL RATS

Sandimmun®, 5 and 15 mg/kg, was administered to 6-week-old female rats and compared with a group of animals receiving only the vehicle. Radiometric measurements of caudal vertebrae and tibiae were performed at regular intervals during the 30-day investigational period. Subsequently, the animals were sacrificed and the radiographed vertebrae were dissected and embedded in methyl-methacrylate for histomorphometry involving computer-assisted calculation of trabecular measurements, and apposition and resorption rates. Blood was also withdrawn for osteocalcin determinations.

Results of radiometric and volume measurements are depicted in Figure 3. Vertebral values were not modified by treatment but there was a small but significant ($p < 0.01$) decrease in tibial volume. This

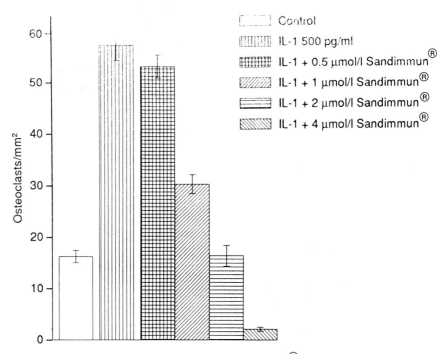

Figure 2 Dose-dependent reduction by Sandimmun® of osteoclast number in calvarial cultures stimulated with interleukin 1 (IL-1)

effect, however, was not severe enough to elevate circulating osteocalcin (86 ± 8 and 77 ± 8 ng/ml for 5 and 15 mg Sandimmun®, respectively vs. 79 ± 6 ng/ml for controls; n.s.), suggesting that tibial changes did not reflect generalized skeletal demineralization.

These results are at variance with data reported by Movsowitz and colleagues[7]. These authors found tibial osteopenia and osteocalcin elevations when Sandimmun® was given to normal rats and only partial recovery on discontinuation of treatment[8]. In spite of these findings, there was no radiological evidence of mineral loss. More recently, Orcel and colleagues[6] have recorded *in vivo* suppression of vertebral resorption by Sandimmun® in untreated rats. They also observed enhanced bone apposition, as estimated by dynamic histomorphometry after double tetracycline labeling. Although no clear explanation can be offered, it is proposed that the different composition of

Day 30

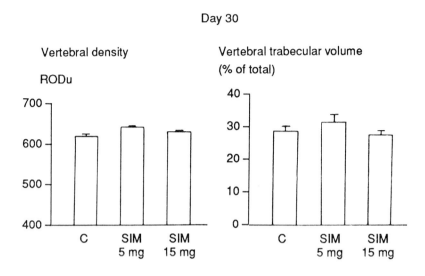

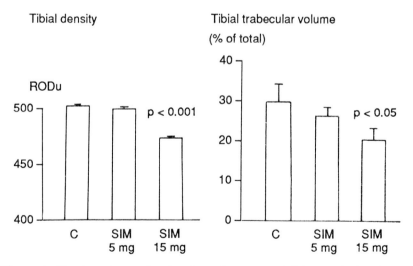

Figure 3 Density values and trabecular volumes recorded in vertebral and tibial specimens from normal rats (*n* = 8 per group) treated for 30 days with daily oral doses of 5 or 15 mg/kg Sandimmun® (SIM). RODu = relative optical density units. Explanation in text

tibial and vertebral marrow, as the source of cells governing bone kinetics, may be responsible for this discrepancy. Indeed, studies to be presented in the next section show that measurements of whole body calcium by a double photon absorption technique failed to show any differences between control rats and cyclosporin-treated animals, strongly suggesting that findings recorded in single bones may not reflect the overall picture.

EFFECT OF SANDIMMUN® ON BONE REMODELING IN ADJUVANT ARTHRITIC RATS

In order to test the effect of Sandimmun® on bone turnover in arthritic rats, a study was conducted in 48 female rats after being randomly assigned to six groups of eight animals, each receiving oral daily doses of 2.5, 5, 10, 20 and 30 mg/kg Sandimmun® or vehicle for 30 days. Eight normal rats served as controls. Surveillance was started on day 1 after induction of adjuvant arthritis.

Parameters measured were: (1) radiometric estimation of caudal vertebral density (relative optical density units = RODu)[11]; (2) quantitative histomorphometry of radiographed vertebrae (controls and 30 mg/kg group); (3) glycosaminoglycan content of femoral condyles for the estimation of cartilage destruction; and (4) caliper measurement of articular swelling. In another experiment, total body calcium was measured at the end of treatment in a group of adjuvant arthritic rats receiving 15 mg/kg Sandimmun® for 40 days as compared with normal controls and arthritic animals receiving no treatment. Determinations were conducted with a Hologic camera using a double photon source.

Results of the first study are presented in Figure 4. As expected, arthritic rats had lower density values than controls at the end of the treatment period (upper panel). Restoration to normal values was observed between 5 and 20 mg/kg whereas 10 mg/kg produced density levels which were significantly ($p < 0.01$) above the controls and the 5 and 20 mg/kg doses. In contrast, a significant ($p < 0.01$) decrease was recorded at the 30 mg/kg level, probably indicative of toxicity. Indeed, the histological evaluation of this group (Table 1) revealed an increase in osteoclastic activity accompanied by a substantial decrease in trabecular volume. Hypercalciuria found at this dosage level (P. Donatsch, personal communication) is also consistent with this observation. The calculated

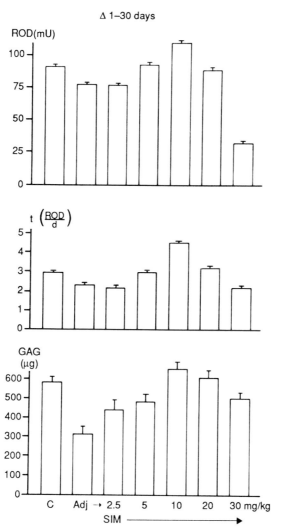

Figure 4 Vertebral density changes recorded in control and arthritic rats treated with Sandimmun® (SIM) compared with the glycosaminoglycan (GAG) content of femoral condyles removed at the end of the experiment. There is a clear parallelism between these parameters. Upper panel: Δ-increment of vertebral density values (RODmU = relative optical density) from day 1 to 30. Middle panel: tangent values of dynamic density profiles expressed as ROD referred to time (d). Lower panel: glycosaminoglycan content (µg) of dissected condyles. C = controls; Adj = adjuvant arthritis; SIM doses: 2.5, 5, 10, 20 and 30 mg/kg (n = 8 per group). Explanation in text

Table 1   Vertebral trabecular volume (%) and osteoclastic activity measured by histomorphometry in rats receiving 30 mg/kg per day Sandimmun® orally versus untreated controls (mean ± SE) (significances estimated by *t*-test)

	Trabecular volume (%)	*Osteoclastic activity (% of surface)*
Controls	28.7 ± 0.7	7.5 ± 0.1
Sandimmun® 30 mg/kg	22.9 ± 0.6*	12.3 ± 0.3*

*$p < 0.05$

tangent of dynamic profiles (Figure 4, middle panel) clearly corresponded with the Δ-differences in relative optical density measured between days 1 and 30. Tangent values also correlated ($r = 0.75$; $p < 0.001$) with glycosaminoglycan determinations performed in femoral condyles (Figure 4, lower panel). This is a rather remarkable finding since there is a close parallelism between restoration of bone architecture and inhibition of cartilage breakdown. A tendency towards lower glycosaminoglycan values was observed at the 30 mg/kg dose, also indicative of toxicity. The favorable effect of Sandimmun® on bone and cartilage turnover was accompanied by a substantial reduction in articular swelling, reflecting improvement of the inflammatory process. It thus appears that the lowest Sandimmun® dose exerting a maximally protective effect on bone and cartilage breakdown following the induction of adjuvant arthritis in rats is 10 mg/kg per day, since 20 mg/kg per day failed to produce further improvement.

These results are in agreement with data reported recently. Thus, the administration of daily Sandimmun® doses up to 15 mg/kg to adjuvant arthritic rats was sufficient to promote regression of osseous and articular signs of inflammation within 10 days, as demonstrated by radiometric, biochemical and histological studies[12]. They also complement older experimental findings showing clinical regression of collagen-induced arthritis following treatment with Sandimmun®[13].

Total body calcium values obtained in the animals receiving 15 mg/kg Sandimmun® for 40 days are presented in Table 2. There is a reduction in total skeletal mineral content in untreated arthritic animals, in agreement with previous data recorded in vertebral trabecular bone[11].

Table 2 Results of total body calcium measurement in adjuvant arthritic rats treated with Sandimmun® (significances estimated by *t*-test) (mean ± SE)

	Total calcium (g)	Hind legs + caudal spine (g)
Controls	9.50 ± 0.33	3.81 ± 0.22
Adjuvant arthritic	8.60 ± 0.17	3.56 ± 0.10
Adjuvant arthritic + Sandimmun® 15 mg/kg	9.45 ± 0.32	4.12 ± 0.22

Significance brackets: Controls vs Adjuvant arthritic, total calcium $p < 0.03$; Controls vs Adjuvant arthritic, hind legs + caudal spine $p < 0.05$; Adjuvant arthritic vs Adjuvant arthritic + Sandimmun®, hind legs + caudal spine $p < 0.04$.

Treatment with Sandimmun® restored mineral content to the normal range. Selective measurements made in the area affected by the inflammatory process (hind legs and caudal vertebrae) showed enhancement of mineral apposition under Sandimmun® therapy, providing further evidence for a positive effect of this substance on bone remodeling.

EFFECT OF SANDIMMUN® ON BONE REMODELING IN RATS BEARING A KIDNEY ALLOGRAFT

In order to test the effect of Sandimmun® on bone turnover in rats bearing a kidney allograft, a group of nine female rats was subjected to bilateral nephrectomy and received kidney grafts from rats of a different strain. All animals were treated for 14 days with a Sandimmun® daily dose of 7.5 mg/kg in order to prevent organ rejection. Following successful therapy, Sandimmun® administration was continued at a daily dose of 15 mg/kg for another 28 days.

Figure 5 depicts the effect of Sandimmun® on trabecular bone density in the transplanted animals at the end of the treatment period. Sandimmun® failed to modify mineral turnover in vertebral and tibial structures, reflecting a lack of action of this compound under the particular conditions of the trial. Examination of serial undecalcified sections (Table 3) showed normal vertebral and tibial trabecular volumes in the treated rats, in support of a normal mineralization process in the areas screened.

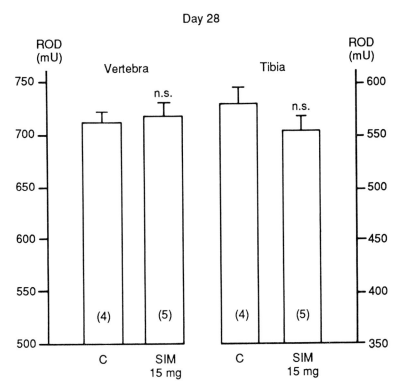

Figure 5 Relative optical density (ROD) of vertebrae and tibiae of rats bearing a kidney allograft, treated with Sandimmun® (SIM), 15 mg/kg for 4 weeks. There were no differences to controls (C)

Table 3 Vertebral and tibial trabecular volumes (% of total bone mass) measured in rats bearing a kidney transplant and receiving an oral daily dose of 15 mg/kg Sandimmun® in comparison with controls (mean ± SE)

	Vertebral	Tibial
Controls ($n = 4$)	31.6 ± 0.5	21.0 ± 0.9
Sandimmun ($n = 5$) 15 mg/kg	31.8 ± 0.7	20.3 ± 0.6

COMMENTS

Sandimmun® exerts its immunosuppressive effect by selectively inhibiting the transcription of mRNA for interleukin 2 and other lymphokines in T lymphocytes[1]. Since interleukin 2 is required for the activation of T-helper cells and cytolytic T cells, Sandimmun® might be expected to act in adjuvant arthritis by inhibiting interleukin 2 production. The fact that Sandimmun® has also been able to prevent arthritis induced through immunization with type II collagen[14] would lend further support to the proposed mechanism of action, since a T-cell lymphokine similar to the adjuvant arthritis factor has been identified in this type of experimental disease[15], suggesting a common etiology. However, a favorable effect on bone turnover by Sandimmun® cannot be explained through its inhibitory effect on interleukin 2 generation, since a primary role in the control of bone apposition and resorption has been ascribed to interleukin 1 rather than interleukin 2. There is, however, evidence for a direct antagonism by Sandimmun® of interleukin 1 actions *in vitro*[9,10], and it has also recently been reported that interleukin 2 stimulates monocyte interleukin 1 production[16], thus establishing a link between these cytokines and their possible modulation by Sandimmun®. The report by Connolly and colleagues[2] of a direct inhibitory effect of Sandimmun® on interleukin 1 release would support such a dual mechanism of action.

More recently, Orcel and colleagues[6] have reported suppression of bone resorption by Sandimmun® in vertebrae of rats *in vivo*, as estimated by dynamic histomorphometry after double tetracycline labeling. As previously mentioned, these findings are at variance with another recent publication showing tibial osteopenia and osteocalcin elevation subsequent to Sandimmun® administration to normal rats[7] and partial recovery on discontinuation of treatment[8]. However, our findings clearly demonstrate that, in normal rats, Sandimmun® treatment resulted in moderate demineralization in the tibia with no such effect upon the vertebrae. No increase in circulating osteocalcin occurred, suggesting that general bone remodeling was not affected by Sandimmun®. Similar studies conducted in arthritic rats and in animals bearing a kidney allograft confirm a lack of action of Sandimmun® on bone turnover. Trabecular volumes estimated by histomorphometry were also reported normal in rats undergoing long-term Sandimmun®

treatment. Moreover, total body calcium measurements performed in another trial showed restoration of bone mineral losses caused by articular inflammation on prolonged treatment with this compound. Thus, differences reported above may reside in the distinct composition of tibial and vertebral marrow, as the source of cells influencing bone kinetics, a subject that certainly will require further investigation. Moreover, measurements conducted in single bones may not be representative for the entire skeleton.

ACKNOWLEDGEMENT

The authors are indebted to Dr L. Miravet, Paris for the osteocalcin measurements.

REFERENCES

1. Borel, J.F., Gubler, H.U., Hiestand, P.C. and Wenger, R.M. (1986). Immunological properties of cyclosporin (Sandimmune®) and (Val₂) dihydro-cyclosporin and their prospect in chronic inflammation. *Adv. Inflam. Res.,* **11**, 277–91
2. Connolly, K.M., Stecher, V.J., Danis, E., Pruden, D.J. and LaBrie, T. (1988). Alteration of interleukin-1 activity and the acute phase response following medication of adjuvant arthritic rats treated with cyclosporin A or methotrexate. *Int. J. Immunopharmacol.,* **10**, 717–28
3. Thomson, A.W., Whiting, P.H. and Simpson, J.G. (1984). Cyclosporin: immunology, toxicity and pharmacology in experimental animals. *Agents and Actions,* **15**, 306–27
4. Stewart, P.J., Green, O.C. and Stern, P.H. (1986). Calcemic hormone-induced bone resorption *in vitro. J. Bone Min. Res.,* **1**, 285–91
5. Stewart, P.J. and Stern, P.H. (1989). Cyclosporines: correlation of immuno-suppressive activity and inhibition of bone resorption. *Calcif. Tissue Int.,* **45**, 222–6
6. Orcel, P., Bielakoff, H., Modrowski, D., Miravet, L. and De Vernejoul, M.C. (1989). Cyclosporin A induces *in vivo* inhibition of resorption and stimulation of formation in rat bone. *J. Bone Min. Res.,* **4**, 387–91
7. Movsowitz, C., Epstein, S., Fallon, M., Ismail, F. and Thomas, S. (1988). Cyclosporin A *in vivo* produces severe osteopenia in the rat: effect of dose and duration of administration. *Endocrinology,* **123**, 2571–7

8. Schlosberg, M., Movsowitz, C., Epstein, S., Ismail, F., Fallon, M.D. and Thomas, S. (1989). The effect of cyclosporin A administration and its withdrawal on bone mineral metabolism in the rat. *Endocrinology*, **124**, 2179–84

9. Skjøldt, H., Crawford, A., Elford, P.R., Ihrie, E., Wood, D.D. and Russell, R.G.G. (1985). Cyclosporin A modulates interleukin-1 activity on bone *in vitro*. *Br. J. Rheumatol.*, **24**, Suppl. 1, 165–8

10. Klaushofer, K., Hoffman, O., Stewart, P.J., Czerwenka, E., Koller, K., Peterlik, M. and Stern, P.H. (1987). Cyclosporine A inhibits bone resorption in cultured neonatal mouse calvaria. *J. Pharmacol. Exp. Therapeut.*, **243**, 584–90

11. del Pozo, E., Gubler, H.U., Perrelet, R., Hager, T. and Wiederhold, K.H. (1988). Non-invasive quantitative estimation of bone density in rats throughout the life cycle and in arthritic osteopenia: preliminary results. *Horm. Metab. Res.*, **20**, 630–2

12. del Pozo, M., Graeber, M., Elford, P. and Payne, T. (1990). Regression of bone and cartilage loss in adjuvant arthritic rats after treatment with Sandimmune® (Cyclosporin A). *Arthr. Rheum.*, in press

13. Borel, J.F., Feurer, C., Magnée, C. and Stähelin, H. (1972). Effects of the new antilymphocytic peptide cyclosporin A in animals. *Immunology*, **32**, 1017–25

14. Henderson, B., Staines, N.A., Burrai, I. and Cox, J.H. (1984). The anti-arthritic and immunosuppressive effects of cyclosporin on arthritis induced in the rat by the type II collagen. *Clin. Exp. Immunol.*, **57**, 51–6

15. Helfgott, S.M., Dynesius-Trentham, R., Brahn, E. and Trentham, D.E. (1985). An arthritogenic lymphokine in the rat. *J. Exp. Med.*, **162**, 1531–45

16. Numerof, R.P., Aronson, F.R. and Mier, J.W. (1988). Il-2 stimulates the production of IL-1α and IL-1β by human peripheral blood mononuclear cells. *J. Immunol.*, **141**, 4250–7

5

Long-term renal safety of Sandimmun® (cyclosporin) in rheumatoid arthritis and autoimmune diseases

M.-H. Pitty, J. Mason, A.-K. Petersen and G. Feutren

INTRODUCTION

Twelve years of clinical experience with Sandimmun® (cyclosporin) have resulted in a well-documented awareness of its efficacy and safety profile in long-term patient management in organ transplantation. Considerable attention is now being focused on Sandimmun® as a treatment for autoimmune disorders such as rheumatoid arthritis, nephrotic syndrome, psoriasis and others.

As in organ transplantation, an awareness of the renal effects of Sandimmun® helps the physician to manage the patient more effectively. The majority of effects of Sandimmun® on the kidney are minor and reversible, and those that are not can be avoided with proper dosing and monitoring. Evidence of this is that only 3% (27 of 938) of patients treated with Sandimmun® for various autoimmune disorders required discontinuation of therapy because of renal functional impairment[1].

The following discussion of renal effects associated with Sandimmun® is based primarily on the extensive data collected in studies of transplant recipients. Whenever possible, clinical trials of patients with autoimmune diseases, and rheumatoid arthritis in particular, are cited. Repeatedly

67

revealed in these studies is the non–progressive and reversible nature of the renal functional effects. The analysis of biopsy specimens presented at the end of this discussion both supports and emphasizes these findings.

THE RENAL EFFECTS OF SANDIMMUN® (CYCLOSPORIN) THERAPY[2]

To understand how Sandimmun® can affect the kidney, it is important to know that this organ is composed of two types of tissue: the renal tubules, which perform the reabsorption and secretion of small molecules from and into the filtrate, and the renal vasculature, whose state of constriction controls both renal perfusion and glomerular filtration.

Functional changes

Functional changes to the tubular or vascular system can best be described as 'tubular dysfunction' or 'vascular dysfunction' which indicates that functional measurements, rather than morphological investigation, are needed for their detection[2].

Tubular dysfunction includes a reduction in magnesium reabsorption, which leads to an increased excretion in the urine and to a decrease in serum magnesium levels. There may also be a reduction in potassium and uric acid secretion, which leads to a decreased excretion in the urine and to a mild increase in serum potassium and uric acid levels. These changes are often seen with therapeutic doses of Sandimmun®, they are reversible upon discontinuation of the drug and are therefore of little consequence.

Vascular dysfunction consists primarily of vasoconstriction, mainly in the afferent arteriole leading to the glomerulus, but also in the efferent arteriole leading from it. This lowers both renal blood flow and the glomerular filtration rate and causes serum creatinine and urea levels to rise. As with tubular dysfunction, vascular dysfunction is reversible, and therefore of little concern.

Structural changes

Two types of structural changes can happen with Sandimmun® therapy:
(1) Structural changes to the tubular system; and
(2) Structural changes to the vascular system.

Structural changes to the tubular system, which can be referred to as 'tubulopathy', can be verified by examination of biopsy specimens. Tubulopathy is found predominantly in the proximal tubules. It includes isometric vacuoles and ballooning within the tubular cells, cellular inclusion bodies that are mostly giant mitochondria, as well as some microcalcifications within the tubular cells.

These changes are very rare and they are only seen with high doses of Sandimmun®, and are reversible upon drug withdrawal. They have no clinical relevance and are therefore of little concern.

Structural changes to the vascular system, a type of vasculopathy, are called 'arteriolopathy' because of their predominance in the afferent arterioles. Damage to the endothelium and smooth muscle layers of the arterioles can lead to vessel occlusion and a localized loss of blood supply. Glomerular collapse and obsolescence, tubular degeneration and atrophy, as well as striped interstitial fibrosis could then follow.

The tubular atrophy and striped interstitial fibrosis associated with arteriolopathy are types of vasculo–interstitial nephropathy. Since this expression is cumbersome, the terms 'permanent' or 'irreversible damage to the kidney' will serve to distinguish it from the less serious, reversible changes to the tubules and vessels.

These changes generally occur when Sandimmun® doses are high. Since they invariably accompany severe functional alterations, they can be avoided by careful monitoring. However, once they are established they are no longer reversible.

To summarize, the functional changes (tubular and vascular dysfunction) and the structural changes to the tubules (tubulopathy) are reversible. They present no danger to the patient provided they are contained within reasonable limits by appropriate dose reduction when they arise.

Only occasionally structural changes to the renal vasculature may occur and these are the results of severe functional alterations. These structural changes to this vasculature can only be investigated by kidney biopsy.

The full picture of all the possible changes to the kidney that may arise during therapy with Sandimmun® is shown in Figure 1.

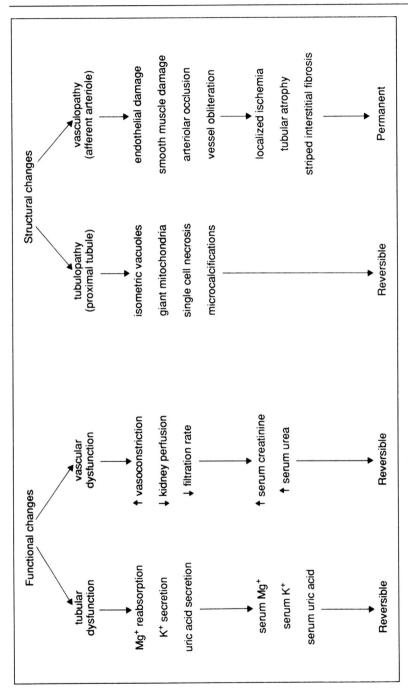

Figure 1 Renal effects of Sandimmun®[2]

STABILITY OF RENAL FUNCTIONAL EFFECTS OF SANDIMMUN® IN RHEUMATOID ARTHRITIS

One of the most frequently used measures of renal function in routine clinical practice is serum creatinine concentration. In studies of rheumatoid arthritis patients, serum creatinine, as a parameter of renal function, tends to increase at the start of Sandimmun® therapy but levels off at a manageable value as treatment progresses. This was demonstrated in a review of nearly 1000 patients treated with Sandimmun® for autoimmune disorders[1]. Mean serum creatinine increased during the first month, peaked after 6–12 months, and showed no further increases thereafter (Figure 2). The mean rise in creatinine at 6 months was 32% above pretreatment levels – an increase that for most of the patients was within the normal range.

This review also pointed out that change in renal function is related to the dose of Sandimmun® (Figure 3). The smallest increases in serum creatinine occurred in those patients whose dosage was ≤ 5 mg/kg per day.

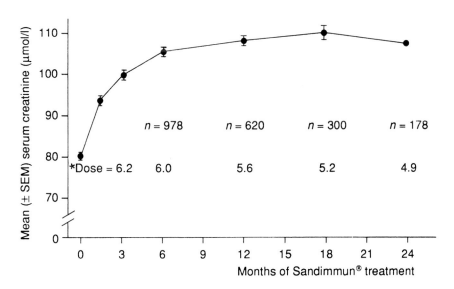

Figure 2 Non-progressive nature of renal dysfunction (measured by serum creatinine) in patients treated with Sandimmun® for various autoimmune disorders. *Mean dose of Sandimmun® (mg/kg per day)

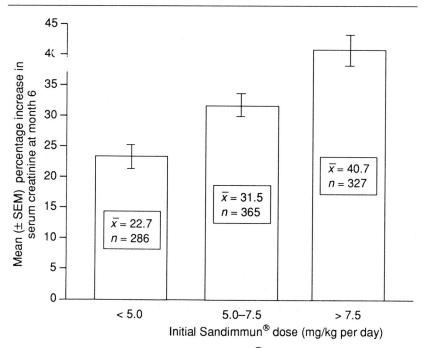

Figure 3 Lower initial doses of Sandimmun® result in smaller increases in serum creatinine over baseline values in patients treated for various autoimmune disorders

Early trials using Sandimmun® to treat rheumatoid arthritis patients often used dosages as high as 10 mg/kg per day. Although effective, Sandimmun® at this dosage produced high rates of adverse effects[3]. In recent years, the stability of serum creatinine over prolonged periods and the almost certain non-progression of renal dysfunction has been demonstrated in rheumatoid arthritis patients treated with lower doses of Sandimmun® (Chapter 6).

This non-progression was well illustrated in the 144-patient, placebo-controlled multicenter study described by Tugwell *et al.* in Chapter 6. The initial dosage was a relatively low 2.5 mg/kg per day, which was gradually titrated according to serum creatinine levels. The resulting mean stabilization dosage was 3.8 mg/kg per day. With this lower-dose approach, mean serum creatinine increased at 6 months by only 27% over baseline. Creatinine clearance, another measure of renal function, decreased during the 1st month and then remained stable during the following 5 months of therapy.

These study results help to determine the optimum administration of Sandimmun® in autoimmune diseases: lower doses (≤ 5 mg/kg per day) produced a minimal and not clinically relevant decrease in renal function that stabilized within 6 months without further deterioration (Chapter 6). Usually this stability of renal dysfunction was attained with dosage adjustment.

The effect of age

When evaluating the renal effects of Sandimmun® in rheumatoid arthritis, the age of the patients must be taken into account. A significant correlation has been found between advanced age and decreased renal function amongst rheumatoid arthritis patients treated with Sandimmun®, especially in patients over 65 years old[4].

REVERSIBILITY OF RENAL DYSFUNCTION

Sandimmun® has a well-known effect on the kidney, encountered in the majority of Sandimmun®-treated patients. However, by proper dosing of Sandimmun® and regular monitoring of the patient, renal impairment can be contained within acceptable limits or be completely avoided; after stopping the drug these effects are largely reversible.

In rheumatoid arthritis, an inherent disease mechanism (possibly arising from nephrosclerosis, systemic vasculitis, amyloidosis, membranous glomerulopathy and focal glomerular disease) and the long-term treatment of the disease with potentially nephrotoxic drugs (non-steroidal anti-inflammatory drugs, salicylates and gold) may already place the renal function of the rheumatoid arthritis patients in an unfavorable condition.

The reversibility of renal dysfunction upon cessation of therapy according to the degree of impairment (measured by serum creatinine), as well as according to the dosage of Sandimmun® has been studied in 210 rheumatoid arthritis patients treated with Sandimmun® in the context of several clinical studies (treatment duration varying between 4 and 24 months), 145 patients had a starting dose of less than 5.5 mg/kg per day. Of these 145 patients, 45 completed 12 months of treatment and, of these, 21 continued up to 18 months and 12 completed 24 months of Sandimmun® therapy. The initial dose was between 1.5 and

Table 1 Mean dosage of Sandimmun® (mg/kg per day) at beginning and end of treatment for all patients ($n = 145$), and those who completed 12, 18 and 24 months of treatment

Group	Initial dose (min/max)	At maximum % creatinine increase	Final dose (min/max)
Total ($n = 145$)★	4.4 (1.5–5.5)	4.1 (0.0–5.5)	3.4 (0.0–5.5)
Treatment completed			
12 months ($n = 45$)	4.6 (2.5–5.5)	—	3.7 (1.6–5.5)
18 months ($n = 16$)	4.6 (2.5–5.3)	—	3.4 (1.1–5.5)
24 months ($n = 4$)	4.3 (2.5–5.3)	—	3.1 (2.4–4.1)

★n = number of patients with an initial dose of ≤ 5.5 mg/kg per day

Table 2 Renal function in terms of serum creatinine (μmol/l) and percentage increase from baseline during the study and after cessation of Sandimmun® therapy

	Number of values	Mean	Minimum/ maximum	95% CI
Baseline creatinine (μmol/l)	145	77	29/136	74–80
Maximum % increase from baseline	145	53%	−5%/229%	
% increase from baseline at cessation	145	29%	−28%/172%	24%–35%
Reversibility, % increase from baseline after cessation				
+ 1 month after cessation	138	18%	−39%/133%	13%–23%
+ 3 months after cessation	115	15%	−32%/147%	9%–20%
3–36 months after cessation	13	7%	−16%/29%	−1%–15%

5.5 mg/kg per day with a mean of 4.4 mg/kg per day (Table 1).

The creatinine was measured (Table 2) at approximately monthly intervals together with other vital signs (such as blood pressure and weight) and laboratory variables. The dosage was adjusted according to changes in these variables. The mean dosage decreased during the treatment period to 3.4 mg/kg per day, this being the last dose before stopping Sandimmun®. The same tendency was shown in patients who completed 12, 18 or 24 months of treatment.

It can be concluded from these data that, in 95% of the patients, kidney function tends to normalize within 3 months after discontinuation of the therapy. Later on, the limited data available show a further improvement of renal function towards baseline values.

This reversibility of renal dysfunction was further documented in the study from Boers and colleagues[5] on the reversible nephrotoxicity of cyclosporin in the treatment of rheumatoid arthritis.

We have seen that the starting dose of Sandimmun® is an important factor for its renal effect[1,4] but also the maximal percentage increase from baseline (Figures 4 and 5) is strongly suspected to be correlated to the degree of renal impairment[5]. Therefore, in the total group of 210 patients an evaluation of reversibility was performed in two subgroups: (a) those patients who had a maximal percentage creatinine increase of < 30% (Table 3 and Figure 4); and (b), for those with a percentage creatinine increase of ≥ 30% (Table 4 and Figure 5).

Obvious reversibility of renal dysfunction is clearly demonstrated in the two groups.

Comparison of the two groups strongly supports the claim that the smaller the rise in serum creatinine during treatment (as a percentage change from baseline), the more rapidly normalization of renal function is realized. This will be achieved by carefully adapting the Sandimmun® dosage.

RENAL STRUCTURAL CHANGES

Results of a comparative biopsy study

In an effort to identify factors that are associated with the renal structural changes in rheumatoid arthritis patients treated with Sandimmun®, one study compared renal biopsies amongst three groups[6]: 25 rheumatoid arthritis patients treated with Sandimmun® (Group I); 11 rheumatoid arthritis patients not treated with Sandimmun® (Group II); 25 sex- and age-matched controls *without* rheumatoid arthritis and not treated with

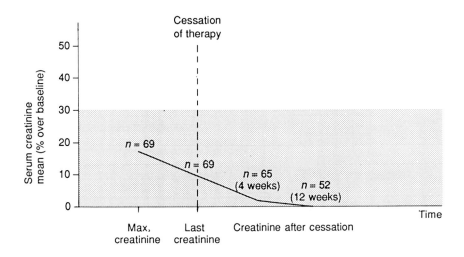

	On treatment		After cessation (% increase from baseline)		
	Baseline (μmol/l)	*Maximal % increase*	*+1 month*	*+3 months*	*+6 months*
Number of values	69	69	65	52	6
Mean	80	16.3%	0.7%	−0.5%	−8.8%
Minimum/ maximum	53/136	−5%/30%	24%/37%	−32%/37%	−36%/11%
95% CI	76−85	14%−18%	−2%−4%	−4%−3%	−26%−8%

Table 3 and **Figure 4** Reversibility of renal dysfunction in a subgroup of patients (*n* = 69) with a maximal creatinine increase of less than 30% over baseline value. Mean age = 54 years (22−75 years)

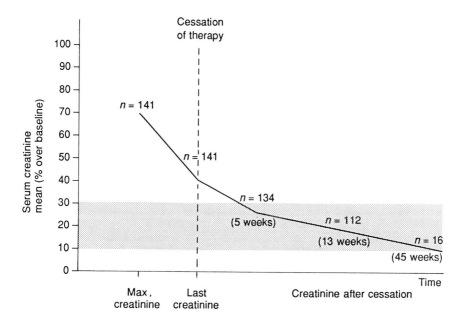

	On treatment		After cessation (% increase from baseline)		
	Baseline (μmol/l)	Maximal % increase	+1 month	+3 months	+6 months
Number of values	141	141	134	112	16
Mean	72.0	69.4%	24.4%	20.1%	11.0%
Minimum/ maximum	29/134	30%/235%	−39%/140%	−34%/146%	−16%/58%
95% CI	69–75	63%–76%	19%–29%	15%–25%	1%–21%

Table 4 and **Figure 5** Reversibility of renal dysfunction in a subgroup of patients ($n = 141$) with a maximal creatinine increase of more than 30% over baseline value. Mean age = 55 years (25–76 years)

Table 5 Characteristics of rheumatoid arthritis controls (Group II) and Sandimmun®-treated rheumatoid arthritis patients (Group III) who had a kidney biopsy*

	Rheumatoid arthritis controls (n = 11)	Sandimmun® (n = 25)
Age (years)	52 ± 4	48 ± 3
	(31–60)	(12–68)
Number of adults	11	24
Number of children	0	1
Sex M/F	4/7	7/18
Duration of rheumatoid arthritis till	10.2 ± 1.5	10.7 ± 1.7
biopsy (years)	(1.4–17.5)	(1.0–39.1)
Duration of Sandimmun®	—	16.6 ± 1.2
treatment (months)		(6–32)
Number of patients on Sandimmun®	—	17
at biopsy		
Creatinine (μmol/l)		
baseline	—	79 ± 4
		(40–139)
at biopsy	86 ± 3	82 ± 4
	(68–121)	(62–112)
SIM dose		
initial	—	4.9 ± 0.2
		(3.3–10)
maximum	—	5.0 ± 0.3
		(3.3–10)
at biopsy	—	3.6 ± 0.3**
		(2.2–6.3)

* Mean ± SEM (range); ** n = 17

Sandimmun® (Group III). The average initial dosage of Sandimmun® in treated patients was 4.9 mg/kg per day (Table 5).

First of all, when comparing the biopsies of the 25 controls without rheumatoid arthritis and not treated with Sandimmun® (Group III) with the biopsies of the control rheumatoid arthritis patients (Group II), the results showed that slight or minimal arteriolopathy was detected in 32% of non-rheumatoid arthritis controls (Group III) of the same

Table 6 Sandimmun®/rheumatoid arthritis: incidence of Sandimmun® nephropathy according to Sandimmun® dose

	Sandimmun® nephropathy	
	Absent	*Present*
Maximal Sandimmun® dose (mg/kg per day)	(*n* = 23)	(*n* = 2)
< 5.5	22	0
5.6– ≤ 10	1	1
≥ 10	0	1

age as control rheumatoid arthritis patients (Group II). Kidney biopsies of control rheumatoid arthritis patients (Group II) had an incidence of minimal or slight tubular atrophy and interstitial fibrosis higher than the non-rheumatoid arthritis controls (64% vs. 16%).

Sandimmun®-treated as well as control rheumatoid arthritis patients had a mean duration of their disease of 10 years.

In 23 out of 25 Sandimmun®-treated patients, the results of kidney biopsies did not differ from findings in non-Sandimmun®-treated rheumatoid arthritis patients. Two patients, however, had abnormalities which could possibly result from Sandimmun® therapy: tubular atrophy and striped interstitial fibrosis of moderate intensity in one case and recorded as severe in the other. None of them had an increased incidence of fibrotic or hypertrophic glomeruli.

The study also demonstrated the relationship between dosage and structural changes. Renal lesions associated with Sandimmun® did not appear in any of the patients who received dosages less than 5.5 mg/kg per day[6]. The importance of minimizing the rise in serum creatinine was also shown: of the 25 patients treated with Sandimmun®, no lesions were detected in the patients whose serum creatinine level did not exceed 30% above baseline[6] (Tables 6 and 7).

Only two patients of the 25 treated with Sandimmun® developed renal lesions that could be associated with Sandimmun® therapy. In both cases, Sandimmun® was administered outside the guidelines recommended for its use in clinical trials. Patient A began at a very high dose, 10 mg/kg per day, and experienced a rise in serum creatinine of more than 100% above baseline. The starting dose for patient B, 6.6 mg/kg per day, also exceeded the recommended maximum of 5 mg/kg per day.

Table 7 Sandimmun®/rheumatoid arthritis: incidence of Sandimmun® nephropathy according to creatinine increase

	Sandimmun® nephropathy	
	Absent	*Present*
Maximal creatinine % increase over baseline	*(n = 23)*	*(n = 2)*
≤ 30	11	0
31−≤ 50	7	1
51−≤ 100	5	0
> 100	0	1

Also worth noting is that both patients were over 50 years of age and that patient B had a 24-year history of rheumatoid arthritis[6]. This and other evidence suggest that patient age and duration of disease may be factors in the development of lesions, but more extensive clinical data will be needed to substantiate these views.

The main finding of this biopsy study was that even after a 34-month follow-up, no occurrence of Sandimmun®-related nephropathy was found in patients whose treatment stayed within the guidelines for safe use of Sandimmun®. To avoid renal structural changes it is of special importance to ensure that the initial dose of Sandimmun® never exceeds 5 mg/kg per day[6].

A similar conclusion was drawn in a study by Mihatsch and colleagues[7], who established that the risk of renal structural changes is minimal ($< 2\%$) if the dose does not exceed 5 mg/kg per day.

CONCLUSION

The majority of renal changes that occur in rheumatoid arthritis patients receiving Sandimmun® therapy involve functional changes to the tubules and vessels. Each of these changes is reversible upon dose reduction or discontinuation of therapy. The only irreversible changes related to Sandimmun® therapy in rheumatoid arthritis patients are structural changes to the renal vasculature. These are rare when the following rules are followed:

(1) Initial dosage of Sandimmun® should not exceed 5 mg/kg per day[1] (Chapter 6).

(2) The rise in serum creatinine should never exceed 50% of the baseline values[1] (Chapter 6).

When the dosage guidelines given above are adhered to, the risk of renal structural change is slight, and Sandimmun® represents a useful therapeutic agent for the treatment of rheumatoid arthritis and other autoimmune disorders.

ACKNOWLEDGEMENT

The authors would like to thank Mrs J. Buonaventura for her expert secretarial help.

REFERENCES

1. Dieterle, A., Abeywickrama, K. and von Graffenried, B. (1988). Nephrotoxicity and hypertension in patients with autoimmune disease treated with cyclosporine. *Transplant Proc.*, **20** (Suppl. 4), 349–55
2. Mason, J. (1989). Renal side-effects of cyclosporin A. *Br. J. Dermatol.*, **122** suppl. 36, 71–
3. Berg, K.J., Førre, O., Bjerkhoel, F. *et al.* (1986). Side effects of cyclosporin A treatment in patients with rheumatoid arthritis. *Kidney Int.*, **29**, 1180–7
4. Ludwin, D., Bennett, K.J., Grace, E.M. *et al.* (1988). Nephrotoxicity in patients with rheumatoid arthritis treated with cyclosporine. *Transplant Proc.*, **20** (Suppl. 4), 367–70
5. Boers, M., Dijkmans, B.A.C., van Rijthoven, A.W.A.M., Goei Thé, H.S. and Cats, A. (1990). Reversible nephrotoxicity of cyclosporine in rheumatoid arthritis. *J. Rheumatol.*, **17**, 38–42
6. Data on file, Sandoz Pharmaceuticals Corp., 1989
7. International Kidney Biopsy Registry of Sandimmum® in Autoimmune Diseases (1990). Risk factors associated with cyclosporine A nephropathy in patients treated for autoimmune diseases. *Kidney Int.*, in press

6

Overview of cyclosporin in rheumatoid arthritis

P. Tugwell

This paper will address the results to date of the completed clinical studies with cyclosporin in rheumatoid arthritis.

Table 1 shows the number of patients with autoimmune diseases (to the nearest 100 patients) treated with cyclosporin as of January, 1989; 600 patients with rheumatoid arthritis have been treated to date.

Table 2 summarizes the completed trials in rheumatoid arthritis to date. As can be seen from Table 2, there has been a considerable variation in the starting dosage used in different studies. It is important that this be taken into account in assessing both the benefits and the toxicity when making recommendations for use by clinicians looking after patients with rheumatoid arthritis.

Studies starting with doses over 5 mg/kg per day ran into toxicity problems in many patients necessitating dose reduction. The open studies using 5 mg/kg or less have continued to show consistent patient

Table 1 Number of patients ($n = 5600$) with autoimmune diseases treated with cyclosporin A, up to January 1989

Uveitis	1000	Multiple sclerosis	400
Psoriasis	1000	Biliary cirrhosis	200
Diabetes	750	Aplastic anemia	200
Nephrotic syndrome	750	Crohn disease	200
Rheumatoid arthritis	600	Others	500

Table 2 Studies of treatment with cyclosporin A in rheumatoid arthritis

Principal author	Trial design	Total no. in study	No. of treated cases	Average dose (mg/kg per day)		Duration (months)
				Initial	Final	
Herrmann[1]	open, uncontrolled	6	6	10	6	5–10
Amor[2]	open, uncontrolled	6	6	8.5	7.8	3
Madhok[3]	open, uncontrolled	20	20	5	6	6
Dougados[4]	open, uncontrolled	12	12	5	5.2	12
Weinblatt[5]	open, uncontrolled	10	10	6	6.1	6
Bowles[7]	open, uncontrolled	10	10	6	3.9	6
Dougados[8]	open, uncontrolled	49	49	—	5	12
Tugwell[9]	open, uncontrolled	20	20	4.6	4.3	6
Forre[11]	open, controlled vs. azathioprine	24	12	10	6.4	6
Yocum[12]	double-blind dose comparison	31	15 (10 mg) 16 (1 mg)	10 1	4.6 0.85	6
Van Rijthoven[13]	double-blind, placebo-controlled	36	17	10	5	6
Dougados[14]	double-blind, placebo-controlled	52	26	4.6	4.6	4
Tugwell[15]	double-blind, placebo-controlled	144	72	3.79	2.5	6 (+2)
Total		224	167			

improvement in the traditional clinical end-points. For example, the study by Dougados *et al.*[4] showed a 39% improvement in the Ritchie Articular Index and a 48% improvement in the Visual Analog Scale, whilst the serum creatinine mean increased from 0.84 to 1.26 mg/dl.

In our own initial studies we started with 5 mg/kg per day but then reduced this by half to a starting dose of 2.5 mg/kg, increasing weekly by 1 mg/kg up to a maximum of 5 mg/kg if the serum creatinine level allowed. With this reduced dosage protocol, patients still showed an improvement in Articular Index by 25% and in pain by 29%, whilst the creatinine level increased by 34% from 71 up to 108 μmol/l. Thus, these open studies showed similar and consistent results that, if confirmed in controlled trials, would be clinically significant. There were two controlled studies without placebo groups. Forre and colleagues[9] compared cyclosporin (in a starting dose of 10 mg/kg, reducing to a mean average stabilized dose of 6 mg/kg) to azathioprine (2.5–3.0 mg/kg). Both groups showed an improvement, with the Ritchie Articular Index increasing by 77% in the cyclosporin-treated group and by 43% in the azathioprine-treated group. Yocum and colleagues[10] reported a study comparing 10 mg/kg cyclosporin with 1 mg/kg cyclosporin reduction to the highest dose that the patient could tolerate with a less than 20% increase in the serum creatinine level. Of the 31 patients, 27 required dose adjustment of cyclosporin due to the rising serum creatinine level. The high-dose group showed a 56% mean reduction in active joints over the period of the study; interestingly, the low-dose group also showed an improvement of nearly three active joints over the same course of time, with four patients showing a 40% or greater improvement.

Three placebo-controlled trials have been published[11–13]. Rijthoven[11] and his group studied 36 patients. The cyclosporin group received a dosage of 10 mg/kg reducing to 5 mg/kg by the 6th month. Again substantial improvements were seen compared with the placebo-controlled group in the major outcomes such as the Ritchie Articular Index (30%) and in the pain scores (60%). The second placebo-controlled study from France by Dougados, Amor and colleagues involved a sample size of 52 patients with a starting dosage of 5 mg/kg (mean stabilized dose 4.6 mg/kg)[12]. Substantive improvements in the Articular Index (42%) and the pain score (36%) were reported, with only two patients having to discontinue treatment because of a rise in the serum creatinine level. In both patients this rise was reversed on discontinuation of the drug.

The Canadian Clinical Epidemiology Research Group has recently completed a 6-month placebo-controlled study of 72 patients in each arm[13]. Based on the experience with the pilot study, the starting dosage was 2.5 mg/kg per day initially increasing to a maximum of 5 mg/kg per day provided the serum creatinine level did not rise by more than 50% or did not exceed 150 μmol/l. The mean dose achieved was 3.8 mg/kg per day. There was a mean improvement in active joint count by 23% and in pain by 22% (Table 3). The results of the other clinical end-points were also all clinically and statistically significant (Table 3). The patients' quality of life improved by a mean of 16% which was also statistically significant. This was measured by the MACTAR Problem Elicitation Technique, a method which involves measuring improvement in the physical, emotional and social functions of the individual patient.

A key question with this low dose was how soon an effect appears. Although in individual patients the improvement appears to be slow, Figure 1 shows that the slopes for mean improvement in joint count diverge from the 1st month onwards; difference achieves statistical significance at the 3rd month. Figure 2 also addresses the issue of clinical versus statistical significance: this shows those patients whose joint counts were halved, an improvement that most clinicians would accept as clinically significant. The number of patients achieving this again increases over the 6-month period. These slopes also raise the issue of whether they will continue to diverge after the 6-month period or whether the magnitude of benefit will remain constant or indeed decrease with longer-term therapy.

There was an increase of serum creatinine of 19.3 μmol/l (27%) (Table 4); two patients out of 72 in the active treatment group were withdrawn on the basis of a rise in creatinine level; the creatinine rise reversed itself within 1 month in these patients. Table 5 shows the number of reasons for withdrawal; ten patients from the active group and 12 from the placebo group were withdrawn for the reasons listed.

Figure 3 shows that, although the creatinine level drops over the 1st month, the subsequent drop is minimal over the following 5 months of the study, which means that longer-term therapy can be considered.

Table 6 summarizes the side-effects seen in all of the patients receiving

Table 3 Outcome measures at baseline and mean change at 6 months

Outcome measure	Baseline		Change at 6 months		Treatment effect	
	Cyclosporin A mean ± SD	Placebo mean ± SD	Cyclosporin A mean ± SD	Placebo mean ± SD	Mean (95% CI)	p-value
Joint count	35.3 ± 12.5	33.3 ± 13.4	−9.4 ± 14.5	−1.2 ± 12.7	−8.2 (−12.7, −3.7)	0.0004
Joint pain	6.2 ± 1.9	6.4 ± 1.9	−2.3 ± 3.2	−0.9 ± 3.2	−1.4 (−2.4, −0.3)	0.012
Joint PET*	168.6 ± 91.0	167.4 ± 57.0	−72.4 ± 92.7	−41.1 ± 78.7	−31.3 (−59.6, −3.0)	0.03
Joint score	55.6 ± 25.6	51.3 ± 27.4	−18.5 ± 25.7	−3.3 ± 26.1	−15.2 (−23.7, −6.7)	0.0006
Swelling count	14.6 ± 6.7	14.3 ± 6.1	−3.2 ± 6.2	−0.9 ± 5.0	−2.3 (−4.2, −0.5)	0.015
Grip strength	105.9 ± 49.8	115.0 ± 57.4	22.1 ± 43.5	1.8 ± 39.4	20.4 (6.7, 34.0)	0.004
Patient global	—	—	2.1 ± 1.0	2.9 ± 1.3	−0.8 (−1.2, −0.4)	0.0002
Physician global	—	—	2.1 ± 1.0	2.9 ± 1.0	−0.8 (−1.1, −0.5)	0.0001
Morning stiffness (h)	3.4	3.3	−1.3	−0.5	−0.8	
Erythrocyte sedimentation rate	48.0 ± 21.9	48.1 ± 23.2	−1.6 ± 13.8	−3.4 ± 22.2	1.9 (−4.6, 8.4)	0.57

*Weighted sum of top five problems

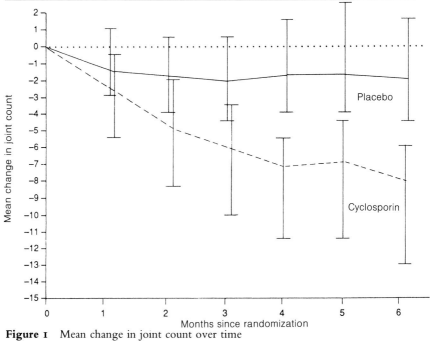

Figure 1 Mean change in joint count over time

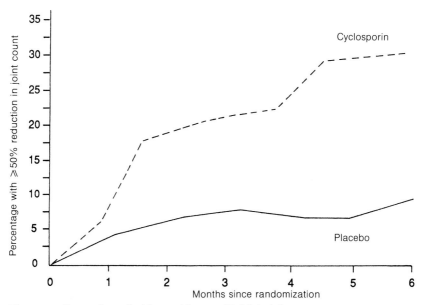

Figure 2 Proportion of subjects with ⩾ 50% fall in joint count

Table 4 Serum creatinine and computed creatinine clearance: baseline and mean change at 6 months

Creatinine variable	Treatment group	Baseline mean ± SD	Change at 6 months mean ± SD
Serum creatinine	cyclosporin A	71.4 ± 21.1	19.3 ± 17.2
	placebo	69.7 ± 14.6	4.2 ± 12.5
	difference	1.7 ± 18.1 ($p = 0.58$)	15.1 ± 15.3 ($p = 0.0001$)
Computed creatinine clearance	cyclosporin A	96.2 ± 32.1	− 19.6 ± 21.2
	placebo	98.3 ± 31.9	− 7.3 ± 18.3
	difference	− 2.1 ± 32.1 ($p = 0.70$)	− 12.3 ($p = 0.0022$)

Table 5 Reasons for withdrawal

Reason for discontinuation	Cyclosporin n	Mean time (months)	Placebo n	Mean time (months)
Lack of efficacy	3	3.8	21	4.0
Adverse reaction	4	3.4	1	1.1
Serious concurrent morbidity	1	2.6	0	—
Death	1*	0.2	0	—
Refusal	1	0.1	0	—
All reasons	10	2.8	22	3.9

*Unrelated to study medication

cyclosporin in the 15 studies described here. Renal dysfunction is more frequently functional than structural and this has been reviewed in depth in Chapter 5 by Pitty. Gastrointestinal intolerances are usually mild; tremor is quite often seen but improves with time without reduction in dose; hypertrichosis is common but few patients needed depilation. Hypertension was a major concern with the higher doses initially used but is less so with the lower doses and, by titrating the dose, blood pressure can usually be controlled.

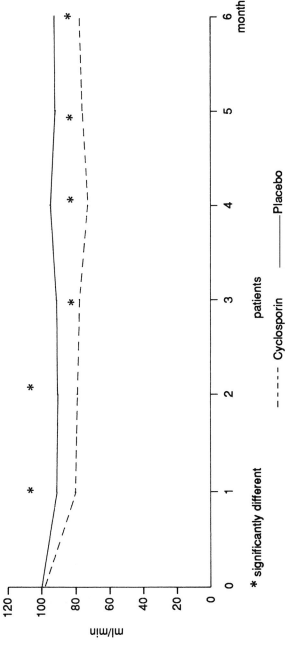

Figure 3 Calculated creatinine clearance

Table 6 Adverse events recorded in clinical trials of cyclosporin A in rheumatoid arthritis. Total number of withdrawals: 40 including six withdrawals for unspecified reason

Event	No. of patients ($n = 167$)	Withdrawals
Impaired renal function	96	12
Gastrointestinal intolerance*	79	7
Neurological troubles†	69	1
Hypertrichosis	52	
Hypertension	32	2
Gingival hyperplasia	20	
Increased liver enzymes	16	1
Flushing/sensation hot and cold	7	
Infections	4	2
Hyperkalemia	3	1
Fatigue	3	1
Thrombocytopenia	2	2
Cardiovascular effects‡	2	2
Rash, pruritis	2	1
Facial dysmorphia	1	
General illness	1	1
Fever	1	1
Basal cell carcinoma	1	
Urinary retention	1	
Mammary hypertrophy	1	
Headache	1	

*Dyspepsia, nausea, vomiting, gastric pain and diarrhea
†Hyper- or parathesia, tremor
‡Myocardial infarction; aggravation of pre-existing angina pectoris

An important question is the issue as to whether to continue giving the drug or to discontinue it after 6 months. It is our experience that the patients need to continue to receive cyclosporin to maintain therapeutic benefit. In the Canadian trial[15], the drug dosage was reduced to zero by a 25% reduction in each 2 weeks and Table 7 shows that the mean improvement in joint count in the active treatment group dropped from 9.4 active joints down to 5 at the 12th month; some patients had dramatic flares. Thus it appears that the drug needs to be continued, just as one needs to continue treatments with other second-line agents such as methotrexate in the majority of patients.

Table 7 Joint count: mean change from baseline after discontinuation of cyclosporin A

Month	No. of patients	Joint count (mean change)
6	62	9.4
8	62	7.14
9	60	7.81
10	55	6.40
11	56	8.70
12	62	5.00

CONCLUSION

The current management recommendations arising out of these studies are listed below.

(1) The cyclosporin dosage should not exceed 5 mg/kg per day.

(2) The serum creatinine level should not be allowed to rise beyond 50% of base line.

(3) The appropriate drug serum levels should be adhered to (these vary according to the method).

(4) Cyclosporin should not be given to people with pre-existing nephropathy, probably not to those with pre-existing hypertension, and certainly not in pregnancy.

(5) Drug interaction should be monitored; it is usually necessary to continue non-steroidals for pain relief but dosage reductions in these should be encouraged wherever possible.

(6) Regular monitoring of blood pressure and blood chemistry is needed.

(7) Kidney biopsy should be considered if the patient is to be kept on therapy for more than a year.

In conclusion, the experience to date would suggest that cyclosporin is efficacious in rheumatoid arthritis with doses in excess of 3.5 mg/kg. Although more controlled studies are needed, the evidence to date suggests that it is as efficacious as other second-line agents such as gold, penicillamine and methotrexate. Long-term nephrotoxicity and risk of malignancy need careful ongoing monitoring, and the place of cyclosporin in the therapeutic sequence awaits more comparative studies.

REFERENCES

1. Hermann, B. and Muller, W. (1979). Die therapie der chronischen polyarthritis mit Cyclosporin A, einens neuen immun-suppressivum. *Aktuelle Rheumatol.*, **4**, 173–86
2. Amor, B. and Dougados, M. (1985). Cyclosporin in rheumatoid arthritis: open trials with different dosages. In Schindler, R. (ed.) *Cyclosporin in Autoimmune Diseases*, pp. 283–7. (Berlin: Springer)
3. Madhok, R. and Capell, H. (1985). Cyclosporine A: a potential disease modifying drug in rheumatoid arthritis (Abstr.). *Arthr. Rheum.*, **28**, (Suppl.) S68
4. Dougados, M. and Amor, B. (1987). Cyclosporin A in rheumatoid arthritis: preliminary clinical results of an open trial. *Arthr. Rheum.*, **30**, 83–6
5. Weinblatt, M.E., Coblyn, J.S. and Fraser, P.A. (1987). Cyclosporin: a treatment of refractory rheumatoid arthritis. *Arthr. Rheum.*, **30**, 11–17
6. Bowles, C.A. (1989). Long-term treatment of rheumatoid arthritis with cyclosporin (CsA) (Abstr.) *Arthr. Rheum.*, **32**, S61
7. Dougados, M., Duchesne, L., Awada, H. and Amor, B. (1989). Assessment of efficacy and acceptability of low dose cyclosporine in patients with rheumatoid arthritis. *Ann. Rheum. Dis.*, **48**, 550–6
8. Tugwell, P., Bombardier, C., Gent, M. *et al.* (1987). Low dose cyclosporine in rheumatoid arthritis: a pilot study. *J. Rheumatol.*, **14**, 1108–14
9. Forre, O., Bjerkhoel, F., Salvesan, C.F., Berg, K.J., Rugstad, H.E., Saelid, G., Mellbye, O.J. and Kass, E. (1987). An open controlled randomised comparison of cyclosporine and azathioprine in the treatment of rheumatoid arthritis: a preliminary report. *Arthr. Rheum.*, **30**, 1987
10. Yocum, E., Klippel, J.H., Wilder, R.L. *et al.* (1988). Cyclosporine A in severe, treatment refractory rheumatoid arthritis. *Ann. Intern. Med.*, **109**, 863–9
11. van Rijthoven, A.W.A.M., Dijkmans, B.A.C., Goei, T.H.S. *et al.* (1986). Cyclosporine treatment for rheumatoid arthritis: a placebo–controlled double-blind, multicentre study. *Ann. Rheum. Dis.*, **45**, 726–31
12. Dougados, M., Awada, H. and Amor, B. (1988). Cyclosporine in rheumatoid arthritis: a double blind, placebo controlled study in 52 patients. *Ann. Rheum. Dis.*, **47**, 127–33
13. Tugwell, P., Bombardier, C., Gent, M. *et al.* (1990). Low dose cyclosporine versus placebo in patients with rheumatoid arthritis. *Lancet*, in press

Conclusions

B. Amor

Sandimmun® as a treatment of autoimmune diseases and particularly of rheumatoid arthritis no longer has the status of just an experimental drug. Data on its efficacy, tolerance and side-effects are similar to those for most of the second-line drugs used in the treatment of rheumatoid arthritis. Data concerning its mechanism of action are probably more important than those concerning the oldest second-line treatment, 'the gold salts'. These data are clearly summarized in the different chapters of this volume.

Nevertheless, there are still questions concerning the treatment of rheumatoid arthritis and some of them emerged during the discussion following the meeting.

The most important clinical studies have a follow-up period of 1 year. It is now clear that Sandimmun® has mostly a suspensive effect. Discontinuation of therapy is followed by a relapse and sometimes a rebound effect. If discontinuation is necessary, a progressive tapering off over a period of 2 months is suggested by Tugwell.

When the efficacy is good, how long may Sandimmun® be maintained for patients with rheumatoid arthritis? There is no scientific answer to this question, but only isolated cases such as our first patient. This man has now been treated with Sandimmun® for 5 years, outside any protocol and despite many contraindications. For the last 3 years, he has obtained the drug by unofficial methods. Considering our guidelines, the treatment should have been discontinued because his creatinine level was twice the basal level and he developed severe hypertension. During these 3 years, the follow-up was performed by a rheumatologist in private practice who sent us the clinical records. Creatinine levels remained increased but stable during these 3 years. Hypertension is controlled when necessary with antihypertensive treatment. After 5 years, the patient agreed to discontinue Sandimmun®. One month later, blood pressure was normal with antihypertensive treatment, the creatinine plasma level returned to basal level, but rheumatoid arthritis flared up. The patient declined our suggestion of a renal biopsy.

As Pitty and co-workers explained, the risk of structural changes is minimal if the dose does not exceed 5 mg/kg per day and if the increase in serum creatinine is kept below 50% over baseline. Consequently, the guidelines suggested by Tugwell, which are very similar to ours, must be maintained.

The efficacy of Sandimmun® has been demonstrated in several autoimmune diseases.

However, it has to be remembered that Sandimmun® should not be used in scleroderma even at low doses, since the vasculo–renal involvement of the disease may predispose these patients to severe renal side-effects with Sandimmun® therapy, as we have been able to observe in two of our patients treated for scleroderma.

What is the effect of Sandimmun® on erythrocyte sedimentation rate? In most studies, Sandimmun® does not influence the erythrocyte sedimentation rate despite the clinical improvement. Professor Panayi, who discussed the laboratory indices of disease activity in rheumatoid arthritis, suggested that Sandimmun® has a tendency to inhibit the production of some lymphokines but not interleukin 6. He suggested the dosage of interleukin 6 in the stored sera of previous studies.

What do we know about the progression of joint lesions in the Sandimmun®-treated patients using X-rays? Dr Forre, in a study from Norway, observed a radiological progression of 2–3% in the cyclosporin-treated group and of 20% in the placebo group. However, this is only a 1-year study.

Dr Tugwell reminded us that the whole area of progression measured by X-rays is something that needs careful evaluation because over the course of the years there is a large amount of statistical noise depending upon the way the erosions are evaluated (joint space narrowing, etc.).

Modulation of bone metabolism by Sandimmun® was studied *in vitro* by Russell and co-workers and bone remodeling in rats under various pathological conditions by del Pozo. In experimental adjuvant arthritis in the rat, Sandimmun® seems to be able to limit bone resorption within some dose ranges (10–30 mg/kg per day). Beyond this dose of 30 mg/kg per day, bone resorption increased.

Are some data available on bone metabolism in treated patients with rheumatoid arthritis? Dr Dougados has seen three of our patients with vertebral collapse and asked if somebody had similar observations or any experience on bone density measurement in Sandimmun®-treated patients. He obtained no answer from the audience.

What are the effects of Sandimmun® on the extra-articular manifestations of rheumatoid arthritis? Once again, the answer to this question is at the present time not available, because these patients have been excluded from the controlled studies. Only anecdotal patients can be mentioned, such as the one observed in Portugal who suffered from severe rheumatoid lung disease and who experienced a spectacular improvement in both lung and joint symptoms.

WHEN SHOULD THERAPY WITH SANDIMMUN® IN RHEUMATOID ARTHRITIS BE STARTED?

Some believe that an early treatment should be initiated when the diagnosis is obtained, before any joint destruction, in the hope of treating patients who have not already been treated with all the other second-line drugs. These selected patients are those that often appear as the ideal patients to those who are in charge of clinical studies for new second-line drugs. Before making this choice, we must keep in mind some facts.

(1) Rheumatoid arthritis begins only once in one patient but its evolution continues for 20–30 years. No more than 1/20 or 1/30 patients are recent rheumatoid arthritis patients. If only these patients are chosen, the inclusion period will be very long.

(2) Sandimmun® has only a suspensive effect on rheumatoid arthritis inflammation and the treatment, if effective, should be maintained indefinitely, even if patients are treated very early, as has been observed in one patient in our series.

Table 1 Kaplan–Meier survival statistics applied to 173 patients. Withdrawal for any reason was the dependent variable

Treatment	Number of patients	Time from diagnosis of rheumatoid arthritis to use of a drug (months)	Order of introduction of drug				Duration of drug treatment (months)
			1	2	3	4	
Hydroxychloroquine	115	32 ± 60†	57	28	17	13	20 ± 26†
Gold salts	142	21 ± 45	105	36	1	0	15 ± 25
D-penicillamine	93	66 ± 92	11	44	25	13	16 ± 23
Tiopronine*	29	144 ± 131	0	2	9	18	20 ± 17

*A thiol compound, congener of D-penicillamine; †mean ± SD

Table 2 Percentage of patients continuing in a given therapy at 6, 12, 18, 24 and 48 months

Treatment	*Duration of treatment (months)*				
	6	*12*	*18*	*24*	*48*
Hydroxychloroquine	63	48	45	30	15
Gold salts	53	35	30	17	10
D-penicillamine	65	40	39	25	10
Tiopronine	88	58	45	45	12

(3) Classical second-line drugs have the same percentage of efficacy on pain and inflammation at any stage of the disease. This is shown in Tables 1 and 2. Withdrawal of one of the classical second-line drugs for inefficacy or side-effects has no influence on the percentage of efficacy or side-effects of another second-line drug.

(4) At this time, 50% of rheumatoid arthritis patients have received all the available second-line drugs after 10–15 years of evolution. Most of them still have an active disease and we need new drugs to cover the 20–30 years of evolution of a chronic disease like rheumatoid arthritis. In my opinion, a new drug must be able to induce partial or complete remission at any time of this evolution and new drug development should attempt to demonstrate that it is possible to alter the course of the disease at any time during its course. We hope that future studies with Sandimmun® will document a real effect on the progression of rheumatoid arthritis.

Index